How to run

BDSM workshops

+

25 topics

Peter Masters

Also by Peter Masters

The Control Book

Look Into My Eyes

Understanding BDSM Relationships

BDSM Relationships - How They Work

BDSM Relationships - Pitfalls and Obstacles

BDSM Relationships - Books 1, 2, and 3

This Curious Human Phenomenon

Imperfect Journeys

ISBN 978-0-9923263-1-9

Cover art by Peter Masters
http://www.peter-masters.com/

Contents

Introduction

In my little part of the world[1], I write, prepare, and run workshops and discussion groups on both dominance & submission and on mastery & slavery. I have been doing these discussions and workshops for well over a decade and generally they get quite a good reception. I think that this reception comes partly from there not being too many folk who delve into the psychology and philosophy of BDSM and who actually look to understand the nature of D&s and M/s as I do. I think it's also partly because there tends to be a bit of a glut in regards to workshops dealing with the mechanical aspects of scenes with floggers, rope, enemas, suspension bondage, and the like.

> See *Definitions* in the appendix for an explanation of the terms used in this introduction and in the following topics.

From time to time I get interested emails from people in other parts of the world about whether I'd be able to do a workshop where they live. I don't travel much however, and sometimes the workshops I run actually only get to see the light of day once or twice locally and then my notes go into a draw only occasionally to be glanced at as I'm rummaging around for something else.

Thus these fonts of the deepest wisdom and insight don't enlighten more than a lucky few because I simply don't travel enough to spread the joy. So, what to do with them? It's a shame to let them languish in a draw when there are

---

[1] Australia—mainly Sydney and Melbourne.

lots of people who might be interested in them and, more, might be interested in participating in such a workshop or running such a workshop themselves.

Well, my answer is the Peter Masters Do-It-Yourself Instant Workshop Kit (i.e., this book).

What I want to do in this book is explain to you how to run a discussion group or workshop, the things you need to know and do, and give you a whole bunch of already-prepared topics to work from. Most of these are topics which I have presented myself and the notes you have in this book are based on the notes I actually used on the day (or days).

You, in fact, become a workshop presenter.

The job of the presenter

The main job of the workshop presenter is to introduce the topic, say something or ask a question to get the discussion started, and then to shut up so that everyone else gets to contribute.

The bit about shutting up is very important. As the presenter, it's your job to get others to talk, to get them to share their views, and—to some extent—to discuss the topic amongst themselves so that over the course of the workshop they develop a deeper understanding. Ideally, this is a process they do mostly on their own. This understanding grows from the topic you introduce at the start and which, if necessary, you occasionally nudge along.

It's very important to realise that if you talk much—even if you happen to know a lot about the topic—then it'll become less of a workshop and more of a lecture. And in a lecture the end result is that everyone only knows the lecturer's views and thoughts. All their own ideas don't get an airing and so the audience is all the poorer for this.

In fact, once you've kicked off a discussion or workshop, the very best thing you can do is *listen*.

When you kick off the discussion you should try not to insert your own thoughts or views, at least not at the beginning. In other words, you don't say, "Today's workshop is on the topic of honour and here's what I think…" Instead you might say, "Today's topic is honour and there are a few questions

I'd like us to consider. Firstly, what is honour? Secondly, how important is honour in a D&s relationship?" This approach gives everyone an open-ended starting point.

As the presenter you also need to function as a discussion wrangler, making sure the discussion stays on topic, ensuring that everyone has a chance to speak, and nipping distractions or diversions off-topic in the bud.

Sometimes things happen during a workshop which will require your attention.

- Some people like or need to interrupt. This can be because they're impulsive and have just thought of something they think is highly relevant, or it can be because they may strongly disagree with what the current speaker is saying, or it may be for some other reason. As the presenter, it's your job to make sure this doesn't happen. Every person who speaks should have the chance to make their point fully without being interrupted. If someone starts to interrupt, squash the interruption, politely tell the interruptor to wait their turn, and hand control back to the person who was interrupted. You can generally do this simply by saying firmly, "Stewart! Please let Helen finish. Then you can can have your say… Helen, please continue."

- Some people might simply be talkers inclined to monopolise the discussion to air their own thoughts at great length so that no one else can get a word in. There's no easy way around this; you often just need to tell them to shut up (politely, of course) so someone else can speak.

- Some of the quieter folk may have trouble speaking up if there is vigorous discussion going on. This can be addressed by encouraging people who want to speak to raise their hand. Keep an eye out for them and when you see a raised hand, make sure you create a pause in the conversation and let them speak.

- If the discussion wanders off track, politely interrupt and say, "We're off topic." Then drag it back on topic with a relevant remark or question. All of the topics in this book have ample suitable remarks and questions as part of the material provided.

- If someone rambles, encourage them to get to the point quickly, otherwise they're wasting everyone's time, not just their own.

- Sometimes the discussion may slow down and need a bit of nudging, and at these times it can be appropriate to chip in your own two cents' worth to get things moving again. Also, and as noted above, in all the topics in this book I have included thoughts, remarks, and questions you can use for this very purpose. Additionally, it can be good to sometimes play devil's advocate and say something deliberately controversial (or even wrong, but with a cheeky smile on your face) to liven things up.

Remember that your role as presenter is to make sure that the discussion or workshop is interesting, edifying, and stimulating for those attending. It isn't necessarily about you airing your own views, and sometimes, for the greater good, you have to be unselfish and specifically *not* speak up.

The point is to get the other people in the workshop to contribute. No one person's views can be valid for everyone, and even the most quiet or inexperienced person can say something which will make others think.

If you happen to be one of the "s" people in BDSM, i.e., submissive or slave, then adopting the role of presenter can be interesting and challenging. This is because you may find yourself in a group with masters or dominants to whom you might naturally be inclined to defer, but as the presenter (or discussion wrangler), it's your job to keep people—masters and dominants included—on topic.

When you do have a mix of masters, slaves, dominants and submissives attending the workshop, it's important to lay down a ground rule or two to make sure things flow smoothly and keep things equitable. A few good rules are:

1. No one is to take advantage of their role or rank to disadvantage anyone else who wants to be part of or who wants to contribute to the discussions.

2. No dominant or master is to "hit on" any submissive or slave (or vice versa).

3. Park your role or rank at the door.

Before running any workshop or discussion, it's a good idea to have done some preparation. This basically means having read up on the topic and made some notes. While ideally you'd only need to say what the topic is and then see everyone joining in in a vigorous discussion arriving an hour or two later at some shared and enlightened vision, this isn't always the case. You need to know a little about the topic though not necessarily be an expert, possibly have a vague idea where the conversation might go, and have some questions ready to ask to help people stay on-topic. The topic notes in this book will help you with all of these.

D&s and M/s

The deliberate focus of all of the topics in this book is:

- Dominance and submission, and

- Mastery and slavery.

It is definitely not:

- Topping and bottoming.

This means that there are some areas of BDSM which are relevant and some which aren't. As a general guide, have a look at table 1 on the following page. If the conversation involves things in the *Included* column then you're probably doing OK. If the conversation lingers more than briefly on any of the things in the *Excluded* column, then you probably need to bring the discussion back on topic because it's starting to drift off-topic, possibly into topping and bottoming.

Topic layout

Each topic in this book is split up into three sections:

1. **Presenter notes** which give you some background or my reflections on the topic. It'll probably be useful for you to read through these once or twice before the workshop,

Excluded	Included
Flogging	Philosophy
Caning	Psychology
Bondage	Power
Sex	Authority
Equipping a dungeon	Control
Wax play	Honour
Piercing	Trust
Predicament bondage	Respect
Fetish clothing	Principles of BDSM
The best BDSM stores	Relationships
Care and maintenance of toys	Wants and needs
Play parties	Role of gender

Table 1: A guide to what's out and what's in

2. What you **read out to start the discussion**. This introduces your workshop attendees to the topic and hopefully gets the conversation started. You might not need to read all of this section out at once, and

3. Some **questions and remarks to nudge the discussion along**. These are things you can say or ask to get things moving again if the conversation starts to dry up. Maybe make a note of the ones you'd particularly like your group to consider.

Part I

Principles of BDSM

Topic 1

Trust

Presenter notes

Trust is one of the fundamental principles of BDSM. It has to do with a conviction or a strong belief in the ability or reliability of someone. There can be two main effects of having trust:

- The first is a lowering of defences. In the world of BDSM one obvious example of this is where someone allows their clothes to be removed and their arms and legs to be tied, clearly in the hope and expectation that very nice things are going to happen, quite possibly to their nether regions, and that they're going to be respected and treated well.

  Beyond the physical, trust might lead someone to expose very sensitive parts of their soul to their partner, fully expecting their partner to value, respect and appreciate what they get to see and share.

- The second effect of trust is that a BDSMer enters into a state of mind based on an expectation of what they think is going to happen. Effectively they are precipitated (or thrown headlong) by this expectation into the first stages of a journey which ends with the satisfaction or resolution of their needs and wants. If they're looking forward to a profound experience with their partner and the initial signals are that they're going to get it, then they enter into a state of readiness and openness for what's about to come. This can be a profound and serious state of surrender and vulnerability.

The depth of this state is going to depend on their level of trust, and this is also going to be a major factor in how much satisfaction they're ultimately going to be able to achieve.

The exploration of surrender—which is equally relevant to masters, slaves, dominants, and submissives because they must all surrender completely to their natures to be fully empowered by them—is often an extraordinarily delicate area. For someone to be able to allow a partner to participate with them and engage with them in surrender involves a very deep level of trust. Without such deep trust the person just isn't going to open up and let themselves be *touched* at all by their partner.

Typically, trust is built up over time and is based on experience.

As an aside, it can also come from credentials. While there are no widely-accepted certificates of submission, or diplomas of dominance, a person can form a certain level of trust and expectation in another person based simply on someone else vouching for them. This person who does the vouching needs to be trusted already.

No one expects that someone else is universally wonderful. Instead, the trust someone has in a partner (or potential partner) is based on predictability and consistency in particular areas. The more areas in which they're predictable or consistent, the more they can be trusted. This trust doesn't have to do with them always doing the same things, but instead means that what they do is generally in an acceptable range.

For example, consider a particular submissive who needs a firm hand from time to time. When they're with a dominant who is strict enough so that they don't become restless, then they can trust the dominant in this "firm hand" department. The strictness doesn't need to be imposed always at the same time, with the same frequency, or even in the same way. It just needs to be *enough* and then the submissive will trust the dominant and feel secure with them. On the other hand, if the dominant sometimes gets distracted by other things in their life and gets a bit slack in regards to the submissive's discipline, then the submissive begins to lose trust in that area.

Similarly, when a dominant sends their submissive off to perform some task then as long as the submissive does it in a reasonable time and reasonably effectively the dominant develops trust in them. If the submissive instead sometimes needs reminding or, heaven forbid, cajoling, then the dominant tends to lose trust in them in this area.

One of the important ideas here is that it can be possible to trust someone completely in one regard, but not in another. This means that a person who is completely erratic or unpredictable in some area is someone we won't be able to trust at all in that area, despite how nice they otherwise seem to be. For example, a submissive who is excellent in all ways except that when she's out of sight her mind tends to wander is not going to be trustworthy in terms of sending her out to perform important errands. For example, if she is sent to take the car to be serviced and she instead buys new seat covers and fluffy dice to hang from the rear-view mirror then she simply can't be trusted for errands. In other respects she might be absolutely fantastic, but for errands, no.

There's an additional element in the trust I'm talking about beyond being consistent, predictable or reliable. It's to do with being able to contribute to getting wants or needs met. When someone talks about trusting a BDSM partner, often they're implicitly talking about their partner being able to help them find satisfaction or pleasure.

It's also quite possible to trust that someone will *not* be able to do this.

For example, a dominant might need a submissive who is open and receptive whenever the dominant is *in the mood*, but the submissive they're with might be a high-powered business executive and she's sometimes too distracted by work and simply may not be able to switch into subby mode all the times the dominant needs her to. Thus, the dominant can trust that she *won't* be available all the times he wants.

Recognising this sort of *negative* trust is important. It's unlikely that a single person will be able to satisfy all our wants and needs. Being certain both about what's going to work and what isn't with a particular partner makes constructing effective relationships much easier and avoids a lot of disappointment.

Read out to start the discussion

Trust, honour and respect are often mentioned as fundamental principles of BDSM, leather and the Old Guard. Today's topic is the first of these: trust. We'll be looking at why trust is so important, and at the role of trust in our D&s and M/s relationships.

Trust isn't as simple as always showing up for appointments on time or always respecting a partner's safeword. Trust is more often about consistency. To feel secure, a person needs to know that their partner will behave within limits which they find comfortable. For example, if they know that their partner is never on time, but that they always arrive between five and twenty minutes late, this is something they can probably accommodate. On the other hand, if as well as never being on time their partner sometimes don't even arrive at all, then this may not be something they can adapt to.

In all of this it's important to consider why trust is taken to be fundamental by so many people. After all, many people's earliest BDSM experiences are at BDSM play parties, and it doesn't require a lot of trust to be tied up or flogged when there are so many other people around.

So, with that short introduction, we'll start with a couple of questions:

What is trust exactly?

When does trust become important to us BDSM folk, and why?

Questions and remarks to nudge the discussion along

- Trust often has to do with expectation. When we trust our D&s or M/s partner, we can enter into a situation or state of mind with them knowing that there's going to be a good outcome. In fact, expectation can start us on the path to that state of mind even before our partner has done anything.

  If we go back to the punctuality example, due to knowing that our partner is about to arrive we might enter into a state of mind, arousal, excitement, anticipation, or expectation for some planned activity with them. If, however, we then discover that they can't be there or that the activity can't go ahead for some reason, we're left in that state of mind and we have to get out of it somehow.

If the state of mind we entered was sub-space, then getting out of it on our own is easier said than done. The next time such a planned activity comes along, we might be a little less responsive due to diminished trust.

In this regard, trust has to do with expectation, about being able to safely enter into a state of mind ready for something to happen. Something similar to the above can occur when a dominant is looking forward to a planned evening of D&s delight and their submissive doesn't show up or just "isn't in the mood". If this happens their built-up expectation is frustrated and the ability of the dominant to trust that future planned activities will be rewarding with this submissive will be a little dented.

- Do we always need trust and, if so, how much of it? Under what circumstances do we need more, and in what circumstances can we make do with less trust?

- Does trust have a role in communication? Can more communication (or less) affect how much we trust someone?

- Trust is often relevant when we're talking about the psychological and emotional barriers which we place around ourselves to protect us. Trust helps us lower these barriers. What sorts of barriers do you lower as you develop trust in a BDSM partner? What barriers do you, personally, always leave in place?

- Does the amount of trust required vary between, say, a dominant and their submissive compared to a master and their slave?

- Do we get a trust issue if a submissive says no to their dominant about something?

- What happens if you lose someone's trust? Can you get it back? Does anyone have an example where they lost trust in their BDSM partner?

- Is it the case that you can lose trust in one area—or not have it in the first place—but still trust someone completely in other areas?

- Is it relevant to think about how much you trust yourself? What problems might occur when you don't trust yourself in some way?

- What sorts of things have happened to you which have caused you to lose trust in someone? What happened to the relationship you had with them as a result?

- How can you tell how much someone trusts you? Is this important to know?

- Does your partner need to trust you in all respects? Does it limit what you can do in your relationship if they don't?

- If you're a master or a dominant, how important is trust in your partner for you? What sort of trust problems can a master or dominant have in regards to a slave or submissive?

- If trust is about expectations, to what extent can trust problems be due to excessive or unreasonable expectations?

Topic 2

Honour

Presenter notes

Honour may seem like an easy topic, but when you talk to people and ask them to actually define honour they can often only answer in terms of examples:

- Honour is doing what you say you'll do,

- Honour is being punctual,

- Honour is always showing up for appointments,

- Honour is being up front and honest,

- Honour is not being deceitful, or,

- More generally, being honorable is when X happens and you respond by doing Y.

The problem is that in many cases these things are only right in certain situations.

For example, if being up front and honest is honour, then imagine you're visiting a friend in hospital who is life-threateningly ill and both their doctor and their wife have asked you to be gentle and not tell your friend the seriousness of their illness. Your friend asks, "How bad is it?" If you tell them that the prognosis is good and they should be out of the hospital soon and you know this is untrue, then are you being honorable? Are you being dishonorable?

Honour is not really about rules of behaviour. Honour is more about knowing the difference between right and wrong in a moral sense. It's about being able to evaluate a situation, determine the right course of action, and then follow through on it. Frequently, the values that you need to apply vary depending on where you are and who you are with. This can make it complicated.

For example, in the world outside of BDSM it's generally considered poor form to have sex with another man's woman. Inside the world of BDSM, it can be entirely appropriate for a dominant to give his female submissive to another dominant for the evening for precisely this use.

Honour then, can be about learning the values and responses appropriate to each group you're involved with. In fact, the term *code of honour* refers to exactly this.

Read out to start the discussion

In the world of S&M and BDSM, honour is often mentioned along with trust and respect as being one of the fundamental principals of BDSM. But what is honour?

Is it a code of behaviour?

Is it a set of rules?

Questions and remarks to nudge the discussion along

- Is it possible to have no honour?

- What is dishonourable behaviour?

- How does honour affect a BDSM relationship?

- In wider society, we sometimes hear about military honour, or professional honour, or "honour amongst thieves". These suggest that there might be different codes or systems of honour for different situations or circumstances. Is this so?

  Following on from this is an obvious question: Is there such a thing as BDSM honour? How is it different to other types of honour?

- Does honour have anything to do with values?

- Is honour measurable? The military can discharge someone due to lack of honour, i.e., a dishonourable discharge. If they can do it, can we say that there must be a way of measuring honour or recognising it? What about in BDSM?

- What values are important in BDSM honour?

- Because it seems that honour, or codes of honour, are different in different groups, would this statement be a way we can define honour?

  A set of rules or behaviours designed to maintain and support the values of the group we're in.

- It's important to consider that in years gone past, honour was a critical part of a person's wardrobe. It is something society judged them on (and often their family, friends and colleagues as well). This suggests that honour is valuable just on its own because it's not something you'd want to lose. Is this true? Is it something you can trade on?

Topic 3

Respect

Presenter notes

Respect has to do with other people. Specifically, it has two parts:

1. Recognising what is of value to other people, and

2. Making an effort to not unnecessarily stomp on those things.

In the world of BDSM, respect has a very important place because we engage in a very different dance in regards to values than do most people outside of BDSM. In particular, self-worth is often in play in BDSM and it's something we need to recognise and work to preserve or even to increase.

For example, in BDSM we can have the elevation of one person above another in terms of rank, often to extremes. Or we can have a submissive or slave being treated as lowly as furniture. When we elevate someone in rank we are inflating them, and when we treat them as objects we are deflating them. In both of these situations, and in all of BDSM, it's necessary for the people involved not to lose the sense of both who they are and that what they believe in has value.

Being treated as an object must still respect the person's feelings and values. It must not diminish them. Instead it needs to be an opportunity for them to express themselves in a way which is authentic to them[1]. It needs to be an opportunity for them to be more of themselves, not less.

In the other direction, a submissive or slave might see a master or dominant purely as an idol or simply as a guy with a whip who keeps them in line. Either of these can potentially be devaluing or disrespectful because the dominant or master may be aiming for something higher, more skillful, or even more spiritual.

This topic has ties into the subject of abuse. It can be easy to put someone down in a way which devalues them (which is abuse), but in BDSM-land putting someone down needs to be done in such a way that it increases their value. In fact, the very same put down can be abusive on the one hand, or life-affirming on the other, depending on the context. In a BDSM context, it always needs to be life-affirming.

So. Respect has to do with values, and one of the challenges in BDSM is how to preserve them.

Another challenge is finding out the values which are important to your partner because these are the most important values for you to maintain[2].

Read out to start the discussion

Trust, honour and respect are typically considered the big three of the principles of BDSM. Today's topic is respect.

An obvious question to start with is: What is respect?

What is it that we actually do when we treat someone with respect?

How does this work in BDSM? How do we treat someone with respect and still sometimes have them on a pedestal or have them crawling at our feet?

---

[1] See also topic 11 on page 57, *Authenticity*.
[2] After your own, of course.

20

Questions and remarks to nudge the discussion along

- How do we show that we respect a partner? Perhaps we could phrase this as: How do we show that we respect our partner even while we're degrading them or beating the crap out of them? And how do we show that we respect our partner when they're pissing on our heads or are sticking mysterious objects up our rear end?

- How does respect tie in with my values and my partner's values?

- How do I know, or how can I learn, what these values are?

- If a submissive is being treated as a piece of furniture, are they being respected? How is this possible?

- If a submissive puts their dominant on a metaphorical pedestal, are they respecting them? Or are they objectifying them?

- Raising someone up or putting someone down can be very powerful experiences for them. What sorts of things can we do in terms of BDSM to enhance this experience while still preserving their humanity?

- In wider society—in the world outside of BDSM—we learn to treat most everyone as equals. How does this differ in BDSM-land? In what ways do we treat our BDSM partner that aren't equal? Does this still mean that we respect them?

- How do we treat ourselves, or how do we present ourselves, so that we are higher or lower (such as in terms of rank or authority) than our partner?

Topic 4

Consent

Presenter notes

There are a couple of mottoes which regularly appear in house rules for BDSM parties and events. They are SSC (Safe, Sane and Consensual) and RACK (Risk-Aware Consensual Kink). Both of these refer to consent. Indeed, consent frequently appears in any conversation about practical BDSM. It goes hand-in-hand with another often-mentioned aspect of BDSM, namely negotiation[1].

Interestingly though, consent is often actually about surprise... or, more accurately, about avoiding surprise. When someone consents to be involved in an activity or a relationship, they don't expect to be surprised later on. In fact, one of the most important things about negotiation and seeking consent can be ensuring that there aren't any surprises further down the track.

When a scene, activity or relationship goes somewhere which one or both of the participants wasn't expecting—i.e., they get surprised—there's a possibility of hurt, offence or anger. Consequently, the best flavour of consent

---

[1] See also topic 10 on page 53, *Negotiation*.

is fully-informed consent because it has the best chance of minimising the risk of surprise.

In this topic, three consent-related scenarios are presented. We look at the role of consent in each of them.

Read out to start the discussion

Consent is one of the key ideas often mentioned when talking about happy, useful and productive BDSM relationships. It's also a concept that isn't always well understood.

In many cases, it's promoted as being about negotiation, about informing your partner, and getting their agreement before doing anything. But is this all there is? Is it really that simple?

Let's look at some scenarios. Each of the scenarios has notable, but maybe not obvious, consent issues:

Scenario 1

> In February, 2012, The Sydney Morning Herald reported[2] on an incident in Oregon, USA, where passersby called police and reported seeing a car outside a market with a naked woman tied up in the back with duct tape over her mouth. A total of nine police cars were sent out to search for the vehicle.
>
> During the course of this episode, the car stopped at several stores while the woman was tied up in the back, and the male driver had done some shopping at each store and then moved on.
>
> Later in the day the driver returned home to where the car was registered to be met by police.

---

[2]Sydney Morning Herald, February 16, 2012: "Pair were just 'Valentine's Day role-playing' as nine police cars hunt down woman seen naked and bound in car"

It's not said in the article, but we can assume, because no related charges were mentioned, that the woman in the back of the car was naked and bound consensually. But what about the others involved?

Scenario 2

> Some years ago, I was at a LGB[3] bar with two female friends for a talent show in which they were performing when a woman came up and asked, "My master was wondering if you were gay?"

There can be a blurring in some people's minds where they see some sort of equivalence between BDSM and LGB sex. But consider the context of this scenario. Maybe there is a higher-than-average proportion of BDSM folk in LGB bars, but would this type of approach be appropriate in say, a supermarket, or in a parents-and-citizens meeting, or at the beach? If the answer is no to any of these, then why is it OK in a bar? Or is it actually OK in a bar?

Scenario 3

> Imagine a male dominant who shows up at a play party. He presents as knowledgeable, has his own toybag full of clearly well-used implements, and offers to flog any female who is interested.
>
> One female who is experienced and who likes very heavy play volunteers. Unknown to her and to the others present, the dominant is a misogynist and while giving the woman a most intense flogging which she quite enjoys, he is muttering under his breath, "You stupid whore! I hate your kind! Take that, you bitch!"

We can ask what it is that she actually consented to. Would she have consented if she knew that the guy was a misogynist and knew what he would be thinking?

---

[3]Lesbian, gay, and bisexual

Questions and remarks to nudge the discussion along

Scenario 1

- What about the person or people who saw the woman in the back of the car and who reported this to the police? Were they involved in a BDSM scene without their consent?

  Perhaps. Consent has to do with things playing out according to expectations and this person or these people left their house that day not expecting to see an apparent sex-based kidnapping occurring.

- We could also consider that the police involved didn't consent to be involved in a *faux* kidnapping, but how far do their expectations go regarding what they might encounter in the line of duty? Is absolutely everything and anything fair game for them, or are there things which even a police officer should not expect to encounter? How should they feel or react if they do?

Scenario 2

- The problem here is that the female slave is explicitly involving me in a M/s scenario by telling me that she has been ordered by her master to engage me.

  In other words, without my prior consent I was involved in a M/s scene. Because I'm a worldly-wise dominant this is a minor thing for me, but what would have happened if it wasn't a worldly-wise dominant who she approached and spoke to? What if it was just some member of the public? Would they feel uncomfortable or confused if they had been in my place?

- How could the slave have handled this better?

Scenario 3

- There's a question of abuse here. Was she abused?

  The word abuse literally means to make poor use of someone or something and so, yes, she was poorly used by this guy.

  Did she suffer any negative effects? From the description, no, she didn't.

  Is it relevant that she didn't?

- Did he, the dominant, suffer any negative consequences?

  We could say yes. His abusive attitude was reinforced. He gets away with being abusive and maybe even gets thanked for the intense scene. This would encourage him on this path and maybe lead to actual grave consequences for another submissive sometime in the future.

General question and remarks

- Consider sub-space. For many submissives and slaves, their first experience of sub-space is intense, powerful, profound, and even scary. It's typically unlike anything they've experienced before. How can they consent to experiencing it when they have no idea what it's like?

- Some people take a "No harm, no foul" approach to consent. This means that if they do something without consent and there are no negative consequences for their partner[4] that it's all OK. But is this a reasonable approach?

- One of the foundations of the idea of consent in a BDSM context is that it is freely given. In line with this, many people consider that changing the parameters of a scene or re-negotiating a scene which is in progress is inappropriate because while under the influence of sub-space or while

---

[4]I use the term "partner" here loosely because if there is no consent, then are they really a partner and not a victim?

27

in an altered state of mind due to pain or endorphins, people can't freely make sensible or rational decisions. Is this true?

If it is true, can't the same thing be said about consent where a master or dominant is feeling an intense need of any sort? If they're in "dom-space" or "master-space", can or should they renegotiate their consent?

- Is consent always important or appropriate? Are there times when it isn't?

Topic 5

Abuse

Presenter notes

In wider society, abuse has connotations of violence. Physical abuse, for example, can be where someone uses physical force or striking to cause pain or suffering in another person. Sexual abuse can be where physical strength is used to take sexual advantage of another. Locking someone in a room or a cage can be emotional abuse.

There's a disconnect here between wider society and BDSM because all of the things I mentioned above can and do occur in healthy BDSM contexts.

In BDSM, we use consent as a guiding principle to help prevent abuse, but is it enough?

In many legal jurisdictions consent is not a defence against prosecution for abuse or Grievous Bodily Harm (GBH). So, if evidence of some vigorous pain play or impact play—such as flogging, caning, etc.—should be noticed during, say, an innocent visit to the doctor about some unrelated matter, the doctor may be compelled by law to report it. Then the simple fact of a bruise or a cut may be evidence enough to convict, even if there was prior consent.

Evidence of a bruise or a cut, or even restraint with ropes or a cage, can be merely a legal convenience, a simplistic way to recognise abuse. But given that many BDSM activities can involve cuts, bruises or confinement, how can we tell the difference between healthy BDSM and abuse?

Often the answer is fear. Abuse tends to lead to fear. Healthy BDSM does not.

Abuse also tends to make someone feel smaller, to retreat into themselves, to hide or to cringe. On the other hand, BDSM should make someone feel more confident and feel that they are achieving the things which make them complete.

Read out to start the discussion

Abuse is a difficult subject in BDSM. In wider society, abuse is typically recognised when there are bruises, black eyes, cuts, or when someone is taken advantage of or imprisoned. But all of these are common in what can be quite healthy BDSM relationships.

We usually can't use society's definitions for abuse, so can we define abuse in a way which is relevant to BDSM?

How do we know that something which looks like it might be abusive, such as when a dominant degrades or puts down their submissive, actually isn't, such as when the dominant and submissive are engaged in healthy humiliation play?

And how can we tell when something which looks like BDSM play is actually abusive?

Given that a bruise or when someone is locked in a cage aren't necessarily good indicators, what signs can we look for to recognise abuse?

Questions and remarks to nudge the discussion along

- Is there a relationship between consent and abuse? Are they connected somehow?

- What are the possible effects of abuse?

- What is the difference between being scared and being afraid?

- Can there still be abuse if someone has given their consent?

- What sorts of abuse can a submissive suffer at the hands of their dominant?

- What sorts of abuse can a dominant suffer at the hands of their submissive? Can a submissive acting like a SAM (Smart-Assed Masochist) be considered abusive? If a submissive refuses to obey a reasonable order from their dominant, is that abuse?

- How can you tell if someone has been abused, especially if they don't know themselves? Are there signs to look for?

- Abuse is quite literally to make poor use of something or someone. In other words, it can be to use something or someone outside the bounds of what was intended or agreed to. Can we use this definition to help us recognise abuse in BDSM?

- Is it possible for abuse to occur unintentionally?

- If we have a slave who says that they want their master to do whatever their master wants with them, is it even possible for the master to abuse them given that the slave has agreed to anything and everything?

- If a submissive or slave forms a relationship with a dominant or master based on an explicit understanding that there'd be regular scenes, floggings, torture, pony play, or whatever, is it abuse if the dominant or master then does none of these things?

Part II

Fundamentals of BDSM

Topic 6

Penetration: doing *to* rather than doing *with*

Presenter notes

One of the things which distinguishes BDSM from most other types of relationships is that BDSM is about doing *to* our partners rather than doing *with*.

Let me explain.

In the world outside of BDSM-land, people get together to go to the movies, to go out to dinner, to play cards together, to go for walks together, and so on. It is the experience they share which is often where the excitement comes from: from the movie they watch together, from the fine meal they eat together, from the game of cards, from the fresh air and fine views they see as they walk, and so on.

In BDSM-land, it's far more about the effect that two people have on each other. The goal is typically to have rewarding, satisfying, and powerful experiences caused or inspired by their interaction. It is about being affected by, or by affecting, one's partner[1].

For example, a dominant and submissive couple typically find their pleasure, excitement and satisfaction in how one (the dominant) exercises power and authority over the other, and in how the other (the submissive) responds to that exercise.

We can call this type of experience *penetration*. Although the term is often used in a sexual sense, it is nevertheless accurate in a wider BDSM sense because what is important in a BDSM relationship is that each person experiences their partner deeply. It is the effect that each has on the other which is important, and typically the deeper this is the better.

It follows that one of the problems in BDSM relationships which are just starting is when the doing to, i.e., the penetration, stops happening and the couple end up merely doing with. We can see this sort of problem happening in the common training scenario. This is where a dominant is training their newly-acquired submissive in their preferred way of doing things. It can be a time of fairly intense interaction and the experience of authority and power during supervision and correction as the submissive learns can be very deep.

What happens when the submissive has learned everything? This is typically where things start to go awry because once the submissive has learned everything, training, the source of penetration for both the dominant and submissive, dramatically loses its punch. It then needs to be replaced by something else, and if it isn't the relationship risks transforming into something which might be merely kinky *doing with* rather than BDSM *doing to*.

Read out to start the discussion

It can be said that BDSM is about doing to rather than doing with. That is, outside of BDSM people do things like go to the movies together, go to a fair,

---

[1]One of the things we might observe from this is that BDSM is more about staying in, and non-BDSM is more about going out.

or go to dinner together. What's important is the experience they share such as the movie, the fair or the food. This experience is what provides the thrill or satisfaction. In BDSM, the thrill or satisfaction comes from us, from how we directly interact with or are affected by our partner. In BDSM, we don't typically look for something external. Instead we create something personal between ourselves based on power and authority.

We can call this *penetration* because what we try to do—whether we're submissive, dominant, slave or master—is to directly affect our partner, to penetrate them and to have them penetrate us.

How do we do this?

How does a master affect their slave?

How does a slave affect their master? Is it necessary that a slave affects their master?

Questions and remarks to nudge the discussion along

- What do you do personally which affects your partner?

- Do you, personally, need to experience your partner? What happens if it stops happening?

- How can you recognise when the penetration stops happening? Is it possible to become jaded? How do you avoid this?

- Are there things which are always effective or penetrating?

- Are there things which are penetrating depending on mood?

- Are there some things which are penetrating but which aren't satisfying?

- What is satisfying?

- What sort of D&s or M/s activities or experiences effect you the most strongly?

- What D&s or M/s experiences would you happily dispense with?

Topic 7

Authority, power, and control

Presenter notes

For anyone exploring M/s or D&s, authority, power and control are often their stock-in-trade.

To an outside observer though, it might seem that a dominant or master is simply doing occasional topping-and-bottoming scenes with their partner using rope, floggers or canes. Or it might seem that all they do is just give their partner casual orders occasionally. Or it might seem like there is no D&s or M/s happening at all and that the submissive or slave is just making themselves available for their master's sadistic impulses just as a bottom would, or they are simply being dutiful by bringing drinks.

Underneath this exterior however, the primary interest of all of these D&s and M/s folk is the exploring, embracing and exercising of authority, power and control. The external things they do—such as with rope, floggers, and even service—are merely the tools they use.

This is very different to topping and bottoming where the same external activities—such as bondage or caning—are instead used to create physical experiences such as pain or restraint which are then internalised by the individual. In the topping-and-bottoming world, authority, power, and control are much less important—or even not important at all—than they are in D&s and M/s.

One of the things we can see is that authority, power and control aren't confined to typical BDSM activities or to a BDSM dungeon. For example, lunch in a public cafe can be a powerful D&s experience for a couple when authority, power and control are being exercised. The dominant may impose behaviours on the submissive which can *flavour* the whole meal, such as choosing the submissive's food and drink without seeking her approval, requiring her to eat or drink only after he has started and to finish when he does, requiring her to address him in particular ways, and so forth.

So, what are authority, power, and control?

In simple terms:

- Authority is the right to use something,

- Power is the ability to use something as intended or designed, and

- Control is being in a position to actually use something.

See below for a more detailed explanation and examples.

Read out to start the discussion

D&s and M/s are about authority, power and control. If we compare D&s and M/s to topping and bottoming, one of the things which stands out is that topping and bottoming always involve doing BDSM-type activities such as flogging, caning, torture, tickling, bondage, and so on.

On the other hand, D&s and M/s *might* include these things but can just as easily take place in non-BDSM environments doing non-BDSM activities, such as in a cafe where a submissive follows standing orders telling them how to eat, drink and behave when they're with their dominant, or at home where the submissive performs tasks and chores as directed and to their dominant's standard, and where they dress as ordered and occupy their time as directed.

Often it's the case that a D&s or M/s couple don't actually care that much about caning, flogging or bondage, but do care about and want to deeply explore and experience power, authority, and control.

So, what are they?

- Authority - the right to use something. This basically means that no one gets pissed off or annoyed when you do whatever it is.

- Power - the ability to use something as intended or designed.

- Control - being in a position to actually use something.

We can clarify these with an example.

If you own a car, then you have the authority to do whatever you want with it. If it's a Rolls Royce and you use it to tote bags of dirt around, then some people might be disappointed, but it's your right to do that.

Having the authority to do whatever you want doesn't mean that you have the power to do it. If, for example, you have never learned to drive then while the car might be yours, you can't actually drive it, even if you're in the driver's seat.

And, speaking of the driver's seat, if you do own the car, and do know how to drive, but the car is in one country and you're in another, then you have the authority and the power, but because you can't get in the driver's seat, you don't have the control.

Of course, substitute "slave" or "submissive" for "car" and you get what we're talking about today.

So, how do authority, power and control figure in your life?

Questions and remarks to nudge the discussion along

- How important are decisiveness or determination for a master or a dominant? Is determination a source of power?

- Are there limits to the authority of a dominant over their submissive? Are these different to the limits of the authority of a master over their slave?

  Are all limits in D&s and M/s negotiated, or can we consider some of them natural limits?

- Where does authority come from? Who decides, for example, whether I have the authority to use my slave sexually whenever I want?

- In what ways can you exercise control over a slave or a submissive?

- If, before they have a master, a slave chooses what to wear themselves, how does a master take control of this choice once they acquire the slave? Does the master get this control automatically when they acquire the slave, or is there something they need to do first?

- What can a dominant control about their submissive? How is this different to what a master can control about their slave?

- Some people dislike the car analogy because it doesn't ascribe any personality or individuality to the slave or submissive. Some people prefer the example to be about a horse instead, with the same issues about a horse being property, the rider/owner having to learn to handle the horse, and about the owner needing to be in the saddle to actually have control. Is this better than the car analogy? Is it better in only some cases, such as for a dominant/submissive relationship but not for an owner/property relationship?

- Are there different forms of authority? Can you consider knowledge or experience a form of authority?

- Does force of personality enter into this picture? For dominants? For submissives?

- What happens when a dominant or a master exceeds their authority?

- Can a master or a dominant delegate some of their authority to another master or dominant when they loan their slave or submissive? How much authority does or can this other master or dominant get?

- Is it the case that a submissive or slave effectively only ever lends themselves to their dominant or master rather than gives themselves?

- Is power a matter of practice? Or is some power innate? What sorts of power are there?

- There's a saying that knowledge is power. Is this true in BDSM? How so?

- Physical strength is clearly a type of power. Is it relevant or useful in D&s or M/s?

- Can skill be considered a form of power? What sorts of skills are relevant in D&s or M/s?

Topic 8

Surrender

Presenter notes

BDSM often seems to be about:

- What two people do to each other,
- How they interact with each other, or
- Their effect on each other.

It's true that BDSM is generally not a solo activity and that it needs a partner to make the magic happen, but what we're all really looking for is an *internal* experience.

In other writings I have observed that people don't do BDSM so much for the pain, the bondage, or the experience of power. Instead they do it for where these things take them. They explore pain, bondage, and power because of their internal reaction to it. They want the pain to do something positive to them. They want a positive reaction to the bondage, and they want a positive outcome to the experience of power.

This positive outcome depends on the person, but the sorts of things we're talking about include:

- A hot n' horny sexual experience,

- Feelings of deeper intimacy with our partner,

- Sub-space, and

- Many others.

A necessary part of having these positive experiences is, of course, that we mentally lower our defences and let the external experiences we're having with our partner effect us internally. This is surrender.

Naturally, we can't let all of our defences down with just any Joe or Jane we happen to meet, but part of surrender is not to them anyway. It's to ourselves. It is surrendering to our own feelings, hungers and desires. It is opening up the door to them so that we can feel them ourselves.

Read out to start the discussion

BDSM is usually done with a partner—with our dominant, submissive, master or slave. What we're looking for through our relationship with them or through what we do with them is some form of internal reaction which is positive for us.

This internal reaction could be:

- Sub-space,

- A feeling of release or satisfaction of some sort,

- Horniness,

- That we learn something about ourselves,

- A feeling of closeness with our partner, and

- Many other things.

But to get any of these internal reactions or feelings we have to open ourselves up them and let them happen. This is a form of surrender. We have to let down our defences.

How important is this surrender to you and how you practice BDSM?

Should a master or dominant also surrender? What do they surrender to?

What do you, personally, get out of surrender?

Questions and remarks to nudge the discussion along

- Are there any other internal reactions or outcomes from this surrender beyond the ones listed earlier?

- Surrender is sometimes called transformative. It changes us. How has your surrender changed you?

- Does our state of mind actually change when we surrender? If so, what's it like and when does it change back? Does it actually change back?

- When can your partner—your dominant, your submissive, your master, or your slave—help you surrender? What can they do?

- When is surrender all up to you? What can you do?

- Should you limit how much you surrender? Why? When?

- In your BDSM, what do you actually surrender to? Is it to your partner? Is it to your own hungers or needs? Is it to your own primal nature?

- Are you afraid of surrender, or afraid of where surrender might take you?

Topic 9

Communication

Presenter notes

One of the important things about successful BDSM of any type is that it is heavy on communication. Oftentimes communication in BDSM relationships is more important than in non-BDSM relationships.

Talking is an obvious form of communication and we see it in negotiations before BDSM scenes. It's necessary that these negotiations be open and honest so that both people in the scene get the most out of it with a minimum of surprise.

During the more common BDSM scenes involving rope, floggers, canes, and so on, and even if there is no actual talking, there is plenty of communication going on in the form of touch, the sound of breathing, and via scents and smells such as sweat or arousal. The pace and intensity of a flogging is a form of communication as are the gasps and sharp intakes of breath upon each strike. The tightness of rope bondage, the way knots are tied, and the texture of the chosen ropes say something.

In activities involving giving or receiving of personal service of any type, how the service is performed, how much attention there is to detail and presentation, the acknowledgement of the service, and so on, are also communication.

And even when we're talking about objectification, the message must be received by the person being objectified that they are simply an object—a piece of furniture, a candleholder, a footrest, a doorstop, or a table. It's simply not enough to give them a candle saying, "Here! Hold this!," and expect them to ascend into objectified raptures. By words or actions they need to get the message that they are regarded simply as an object and this message must be *heard* loud and clear or else the effect is lost.

An important factor in BDSM communication is lack of ambiguity. It's often the case that there isn't an opportunity for clarification or for asking, "What did you mean?" in response to some word or action. A submissive who is tied and gagged or a slave who has been given speech restrictions may not be able to ask and so what their dominant or master tells them must be crystal clear the first time. Likewise, a dominant or top may only get one chance to correctly interpret a gasp or whimper and so how a tied-and-gagged submissive expresses themselves can be a big influence on how well a scene progresses.

Communication also creates expectations and so openness and clarity often set the stage for what is going to come. Getting communication wrong can lead to false expectations and disappointment, or worse.

By definition, relationships are about *relating*, and relating is about connecting and communicating. In BDSM scenes, the time-frame for communicating is fairly short. It's limited, clearly, by the scene itself. In relationships, the time-frame is much longer and this can change the nature of the communication. Some things can be allowed to take longer to express and there is perhaps more opportunity for subtlety.

The point is though, that *it's very important*.

Read out to start the discussion

We can say that communication is about getting an idea from inside one person's head into another's. In the world of BDSM we often need to be much more careful about doing this than we would in a non-BDSM context.

For example, if a master is directing his slave using hand signals which he has trained her to recognise, the depth of feelings of control and surrender they both feel from this is going to be significantly deflated if the slave isn't getting the message and suddenly needs to break her silence and say, "Eh? What?"

Negotiation—which is heavily reliant on communication—is a common element prior to many BDSM activities and it serves to create positive expectations and eliminate unfortunate surprises. Getting negotation right is often vital to good BDSM.

In short: Communication is about getting a message across, and it doesn't need to be verbal.

What ways do we communicate during our BDSM scenes and in our BDSM relationships which are different to what we might see in non-BDSM contexts?

Apart from words and gestures, how else do we communicate?

Questions and remarks to nudge the discussion along

- Do dominants communicate differently than submissives?
- Are there any things special which a submissive or slave needs to do when they have something to say to their master or dominant?
- Does ambiguity have a place in communication? Are there times when it's useful or productive to be ambiguous? Can the uncertainty it creates be useful, say in a mind-fuck?
- Can communication impact the authority dynamic between a master and a slave, or between a dominant and a submissive?
  - How can good communication reinforce the authority dynamic?
  - How can poor communication harm the authority dynamic?
- Is omission ever appropriate when communicating? If so, when? And when is it definitely bad to omit something?
- What message or messages might a slave send by how they perform a service for their master? That they're keen? That they're bored? That they're dissatisfied?

51

- Does the nature of communication differ between what we might do in a one-off BDSM scene and what we might do in a long-term relationship?

Topic 10

Negotiation

Presenter notes

For a top about to embark on a scene with a new submissive or bottom, negotiating with their new partner about what they're going to do or not do is typically seen as vital. This negotiation goes hand-in-hand with getting the submissive's informed consent to proceed[1].

Negotiation typically involves things such as describing in detail what the top has in mind, learning about any limits the submissive might have, agreeing on a safeword, and so on. It creates an expectation in both the top and the submissive about what each is going to do, and what each is wanting to get out of their scene together.

Negotiation is generally an intellectual or rational exercise. It's supposed to be where reasoned judgement informs both the choices suggested and the offers accepted. Each person considers their well-being and their goals as part of this, even if it's just to have a quick orgasm. It is, in a way, a form of protection to ensure that scenes and activities don't go to an inappropriate

---

[1] See also topic 4 on page 23, *Consent*.

place. Importantly, negotiation protects the tops, dominants and masters just as much as the bottoms, submissives and slaves.

Negotiation is understandable in the context I mentioned above where two people who don't know each other want to do a scene together. It's certainly appropriate in the case of a top and a bottom for them to negotiate before every scene, even if they do scenes together all the time, and even if the negotiation is only a very brief, "How about I tie you up and flog your balls?," which is answered with, "OK. Sweet!"

One point about negotiation is that by negotiating you're trying *not* to disempower your partner by making choices for them without their consent. But how does this work in D&s or M/s relationships where a very real goal of a submissive or slave is for their partner—their dominant or master—to have power over them? In this case, wouldn't negotiation defeat the purpose because disempowerment, at least in some ways, is precisely the point of D&s and M/s?

The point I made above about negotiating being an intellectual exercise is an important one. It's generally seen as a poor idea to try to renegotiate a scene after the scene has started. This is because either the top, the submissive, or both might be under the influence of sub-space, lust, hormones or adrenaline and may not be able to make the same sort of sensible choices they were able to make before the scene. In other words, during a scene one or both particpants may not be as rational or able to think as clearly as they could before the scene. This means that they may not even be competent to renegotiate.

Read out to start the discussion

Negotiation is a process we go through with our partner so that we both have an understanding of each others':

1. Goals for a scene and what we each intend to contribute, and

2. Limits—such as physical, medical, sexual or emotional.

The end result is that both of us can give informed consent to what is about to happen.

Additionally, one effect of negotiation is that neither of the two people concerned are disempowered by the other. Everything is supposed to be open and above board and choices should be made freely.

This might be OK when we're talking about tops and bottoms who only do mutually-agreed scenes together, but is it OK with dominants and submissives, or with masters and slaves?

Isn't it the case that a submissive hands over at least some authority to their dominant, and that a slave effectively hands over all authority to their master? Shouldn't this mean that negotiation in their cases is unnecessary? Can't the dominant or master then just make decisions unilaterally?

Questions and remarks to nudge the discussion along

- Are there simple ways to get negotiation right? What is "right"?

- Does negotiating with a submissive disempower a dominant?

- Is it the case that in D&s and M/s relationships negotiation should only occur once, and only at the beginning of the relationship?

- Are there some things which should always be negotiated? Even in a long-term relationship?

- Are there some things which shouldn't be negotiated?

- Does negotiation spoil the experience for submissives or slaves? Does needing to consent spoil it?

- Is negotiation equally appropriate for topping and bottoming, D&s, and M/s?

- In longer-term D&s or M/s relationships, should opportunities for renegotiation be deliberately included and planned?

- Does negotiation lose relevance over time for a couple? Does knowing your partner well obviate any need for negotiation?

- It's generally considered inappropriate to reconsider the terms of a scene, or to renegotiate a scene, after the scene has started. Why is this?

Topic 11

Authenticity

Presenter notes

The words "authentic" and "authenticity" get dropped into conversations about BDSM from time to time and it's probably useful to consider what they mean in a BDSM context.

We can start by considering an area of daily life where we come across the word "authentic" frequently and this is when talking about cooked or prepared food. If we see a restaurant advertising "authentic Cajun cooking", what does this mean? If we order gumbo in a genuine Cajun restaurant, what is the difference between what we get there and what's labelled "Cajun gumbo" in a cheap market somewhere? Is there more gumbo-ness in what we get in a Cajun restaurant? If we go to a nice cafe which has a variety of styles of cooking on the menu—such as Chinese, Middle-Eastern, and Mid-Western USA—and one of their offerings is a bowl of Cajun gumbo, how do we know it's authentically Cajun? Does it matter?

Why do we look for authenticity? When we look for authentic Cajun gumbo is it because plain ol' gumbo offends the aesthetic? Is it because we want a genuine Cajun experience? Is it simply because we want something to stave off hunger and real Cajun exactly fits the bill as far as our stomach is concerned?

Is it maybe because we're looking for a real experience of something rather than someone's impression of it?

Let's turn our attention now to something closer to our BDSM home, namely flogging. When a submissive or slave receives a flogging, are they looking for just flogging? Or are they instead looking for flogging *plus* the psychological experience of placing themselves in the hands of someone who will take control of them for the duration of the flogging scene and then hand back control when the scene is over? On the face of it, both of these may be called domination but only one might be called *authentic* domination. The other is merely a flogging. It's just like food which looks Cajun. It might be fantastic food, just as a flogging might be a fantastic, well-executed flogging, but it's only Cajun-like, just as the flogging might only be domination-like.

Maybe what we can say is that authenticity is about presenting yourself accurately, reliably and without pretense. What is on offer is exactly what is advertised. What's written on the box is what's inside.

There's a cost involved in being authentic. It means that you don't inflate what you are and that you present yourself unambiguously so that other people seeing you or meeting you can't imagine that you're any different than you are. You don't get the benefit of ambiguity or the benefit of other people's fantasies about you. If you go through your BDSM life happily just flogging and fucking, then it's like wearing a T-shirt to BDSM events which prominently says, "Dude with flogger. Will flog for sex." No one can get the wrong idea.

So being authentic is about being up-front and honest. But to be up-front and honest with others, you first need to be up-front and honest with yourself. You need full awareness of what's going on, and full awareness of what is motivating you and the reasons why you are making the choices that you are making. Note that it can be remarkably easy to justify any choice and come up with plausible-sounding excuses for making it, but justification isn't necessarily a reason. Sounding plausible doesn't mean it's honest.

Read out to start the discussion

The words "authentic" and "authenticity" get mentioned in regards to BDSM from time to time. What do they mean?

If I say that I am an authentic dominant, or an authentic submissive, what does that say about me?

If I say that the BDSM I practice with my partner or partners is authentic, what does that mean and how does it differ from inauthentic BDSM?

Questions and remarks to nudge the discussion along

- Is authenticity about trust?

- Is authenticity about being open and honest about your intent and what you want to get?

- Is being purposeful related to being authentic?

- Is transparency involved in authenticity? Can you be authentic without being transparent? Do you always need to show all the cards you're holding?

  Can we talk about:

  - Transparency of intentions, both to yourself and to others?
  - Transparency about your wants and needs?
  - Transparency about what your partner is going to get out of their relationship with you?

- Is authenticity about being honest with yourself?

- Is authenticity about not sending mixed messages? Is it about being direct and to the point in what you say and do?

- Is authenticity related to learning about yourself and enlightenment?

- Is authenticity a goal we should be aiming for? Can we get good stuff out of D&s or M/s without it?

- Is it true that topping and bottoming, particularly sensation- or pain-based play, don't need authenticy, but D&s and M/s do need it?

- What limits do lack of authenticity impose?

- What doors does authenticity open?

- Does authenticity have a down side?

- If we consider that authenticity is a desirable thing, why aren't more people authentic?

Topic 12

Pain and suffering

Presenter notes

Pain and suffering, in one form or another, are frequent elements in BDSM. In fact, it's hard to imagine a BDSM play party without them.

Why is this?

I would suppose that it's rather subjective why they are so prevalent. One reason might be that it's because there's an intensity automatically involved with both of them, and intensity is often the name of the game in BDSM.

We tend to think of them in physical terms, such as physical pain or physical suffering, but there are other forms. We might talk about frustration, such as in predicament bondage, or even deprivation of liberty, such as in ordinary rope bondage, as being forms of suffering even though there might not be any physical pain at all. Even tickling can be a form of suffering or torture.

Sometimes, too, when it is physical, there's a focus on parts of the body typically associated with sex, such as nipple torture, cock-and-ball torture, labia clamps, ice dildos, and so on. What is so special about pain in these places?

I like to think that there are two main answers to *why pain and suffering?*

The first is that they can be an intense *shared* experience between two people, and this can be both personally profound and also very effective in promoting a deep and intimate relationship.

The second is that when pain is strong enough it can compel surrender, and surrender is often a goal for people's BDSM activities[1].

Read out to start the discussion

Pain and suffering, in one form or another, are frequent elements in BDSM. In fact, it's hard to imagine a BDSM play party without them.

But are they actually required?

Would you be able to have an effective D&s or M/s relationship without any pain or suffering at all?

What if we're not just talking about physical pain or suffering?

Questions and remarks to nudge the discussion along

- Why is it that parts of the body associated with sex are common targets for inflicting pain, such as nipple torture or cock-and-ball torture? Is it because they're more sensitive? Or is it something else?

- Is the deprivation of liberty which someone experiences in bondage a form of suffering?

- What role do pain or suffering have in D&s or M/s?

- When do pain or suffering help or reinforce D&s or M/s?

- When do they hinder or fracture them? Can pain or suffering be mis-applied?

---

[1] See also topic 8 on page 45, *Surrender.*

- Are pain and suffering so important because they can be turned up in intensity to such an extent that they can't be resisted and that they then compel surrender? Is it, in fact, surrender that some people are looking for rather than the pain or suffering *per se*?

- Is there artistry involved in the inflicting of pain?

- Does the restraint a slave experiences through following orders, or through required behaviour and protocols, create a form of suffering? Wouldn't they be better off doing whatever they want?

Part III

General topics

Topic 13

What sorts of D&s and M/s relationships can we have?

Presenter notes

D&s and M/s relationships aren't a one-size-fits-all proposition. Some people like having an almost-casual D&s relationship where the dominant operates mostly as a guide. Some look for objectification. Other people like something more formal with the slave's or submissive's behaviour dictated by strict protocols. Observing this range prompts the questions:

- How many different types of D&s or M/s relationship can there be?

- How do we know which one is right for us?

Before we can answer these, we also need to consider what a relationship is. It can be very tempting to think that it's about living together, but is this true or even reasonable in terms of BDSM? Some submissives visit a professional dominatrix from time to time and they might have a long-term relationship though they clearly don't live together. Even for people who live together, their D&s might not be *on* all the time. They may just get into gear when one or the other feels a want or need for some D&s action. The rest of the time they may just live ordinary, non-BDSM lives.

The answer for a lot of this is going to depend on why each person is pursuing a D&s or M/s relationship. When *being* a dominant or a submissive gives the person a feeling of being complete or whole then being in a 24/7 D&s relationship is probably indicated. For someone who instead uses their D&s activities as an outlet, then rather than try for always-on D&s with their partner they may be better off just engaging in D&s when they feel the want or need.

On top of this, the nature of what satisfies each person is going to be an important factor. If the slave or submissive feels a need to submerge their personality for a time then maybe being property for an owner is the way to go. Or, if they feel a deep need to be useful, then being in some sort of service, even formal service, might be right for them. The wants or needs of the dominant, of course, need to be complementary. A dominant who simply wants to focus exclusively on their own needs or projects might be best served by a partner who is property, while a master who is aiming to create a team with himself (or herself) as the boss could find a service-oriented submissive to be best for them.

Read out to start the discussion

D&s and M/s relationships aren't a one-size-fits-all proposition. When we look around the BDSM scene or community we can see people who have been together for a long time who might have something very casual and who roll out the D&s only occasionally, and we might see others who have been through a formal collaring ceremony, who address each other as "Sir" and "girl" all the time, and who "walk the talk" as much as they possibly can.

This begs the questions:

What types of D&s or M/s relationships can there be?

Can they be full-on all the time?

How much contact do the two people need to have? Do they need to live together? Can it be entirely casual or on an as-needed basis?

Questions and remarks to nudge the discussion along

- Are all types of D&s or M/s relationship viable in the long term? For example, can someone simply be an object for their partner for years? Does a submissive ever get tired of being submissive? Does service ever end?

- How does role play fit in?

    - Is there a place for role play in D&s or M/s?
    - Is role play workable as a basis for a relationship in the long term?

- Are there pathways for progress?

    - Can and should the nature of the D&s or M/s change over time?
    - Should it be planned?
    - In particular, if a relationships starts out with a trainer/trainee flavour, how should it evolve as the training ends?

- Is being service-oriented necessary for a submissive or slave?

- Is a dominant or master responsible for the wants, needs, and well-being of their partner?

    - Always? What if the submissive's role is "object"? Should an object get maintenance?
    - Is this responsibility the same in every relationship?
    - Is a slave or submissive responsible for the wants, needs, and well-being of their master or dominant?

Topic 14

The Boat

Presenter notes

This topic involves a little story about a boat. The short form of the story is that the boat is built by a slave and the slave's friend. Once it's finished, for a time they both use the boat, but there then comes a day when the slave's master orders the slave to destroy the boat. The slave does this. End of story.

The topic can raise a number of questions:

- In strictly legal terms one could argue that the slave is guilty of destruction of property. The boat isn't theirs (or their master's) to destroy because it's actually shared property. Should the police be called? Should the slave be prosecuted?

- As the master knew beforehand that the boat was going to be built, was it fair or reasonable of them to order the boat to be destroyed?

- Should the slave have refused to destroy the boat?

- How should the slave's friend react to the destruction of the boat?

- And many others.

Fundamental BDSM principles, such as trust, honour, and respect can also, and probably should, pop their heads up in this discussion.

There are a few different viewpoints which may appear during this workshop:

1. The slave has clearly done something illegal and the police should be called,

2. The master shouldn't have done this and the slave should break up with them,

3. The slave shouldn't have obeyed, and

4. The slave's friend should dump the slave as a friend because destroying shared property is unacceptable.

An important consideration in this is how important is the boat to the friend? How much value do they associate with owning or sharing the boat with their [slave] friend?

The story can also be considered to be a metaphor for what happens when a master decides to order their slave to end or change a friendship which the slave has with a third party. A relationship is also something which is built over time and which is owned by both the slave and their friend.

Read out to start the discussion

Consider this story:

> Some time ago, a friend and I were at a barbecue in a park next to one of the rivers in Sydney[1]. This friend of mine was a slave and he had a master who lived in Melbourne[2].
>
> While we were sitting there watching boats go past, my friend suddenly said, "How about we build a boat?" That might sound a

---

[1] A major city on the east coast of Australia

[2] Another major Australian city, approximately 1000 km or 600 miles south of Sydney

bit strange, but he was good with his hands, was always building things out of wood—tables, chairs, and the occasional piece of dungeon furniture—and I was brought up by a tradesman father who had built the family house from scratch when things were very tight, so the idea of building something like this wasn't too radical for either of us.

So we talked about it and we eventually decided that we could aim for something modest with maybe four berths so we could stay the night in it if we wanted, and make it strictly for cruising up and down the river.

He asked his master for permission and his master said, "Go for it."

We managed to scrounge a large-enough corner of a boat shed and bought ourselves a bunch of wood. We worked on the boat at least one day most weekends, and sometimes one or both of us would put in some hours during the week as well.

After more than two years it was done. It had been hard work, and we both had had to learn an awful lot because a boat was something way bigger than either of us had ever built, but with occasional advice from others we finished it and it wasn't half bad. And, in fact, it was better than that because when we launched it, it floated, didn't roll over, and didn't leak (much) at all.

There's a lot of satisfaction which comes from building something yourself and this was the first thing either of us had built like this and we were both quite chuffed.

Anyway, as time and weather permitted, we would take the boat out, then tie up somewhere nice, light our little propane barbecue, have lunch, enjoy the view and talk about extremely profound things (like the weather).

Much time passed and then one day my friend's master told him he didn't want him to have anything to do with the boat any more and ordered him to destroy it. My friend went straight down to the boat shed and demolished the boat. All that was left were piles of wood and a stack of fittings. . . and our propane barbecue.

Thoughts or comments?

Questions and remarks to nudge the discussion along

- Should the police have been called?

- While you might argue that the master should not have ordered their slave to destroy the boat, what would be the cost to the slave of this disobedience?[3] I'm not talking about possible punishment by the master, such as caning, but about the personal cost of disobedience. Many slaves seek to be the most pleasing and obedient they can, committed to serving their master. What price is it to them if they feel compelled to disobey? Does this put them on a path they don't want to be on where they start questioning their master?

- Is the master respecting their slave's friend?

- Should the master (or the slave) compensate the slave's friend for the loss of the boat?

- How important in all of this is the value of the boat to the slave's friend? If the most valuable thing for the friend was the experience and challenge of building the boat in the first place, is it still so important that the slave destroyed it?

- How important is the friend's understanding of the slave's commitment to obedience? Should the friend continue to see their slave friend in a positive light and instead think that it's the master who is poorly equipped in the honour department?

- What happens if we're not talking about a boat but if we're talking about a relationship, a friendship which the slave and their friend have built up over time? Can or should the master order the relationship terminated in any circumstances? What happens to the slave's friend if this is done? Don't they lose their friend, the slave, all on the whim of the distant master? Is this fair?

---

[3]See also topic 21 on page 103, *The cost to a slave of disobeying.*

Topic 15

Holistic BDSM

Presenter notes

I was at a workshop recently where the presenter was discussing various aspects of BDSM. One of the attendees commented that the presenter seemed to have a very holistic view of BDSM.

This is an important observation.

BDSM is not just doing the same things the same way with every BDSM partner you have. For BDSM activities or relationships to be most effective they need to be considered, planned and carried out in the context of each individual involved. In other words, holistically. Doing the same, cookie-cutter style BDSM with every partner may be a way of getting some superficial jollies but it's unlikely to be deeply satisfying.

BDSM also doesn't or needn't just touch one aspect of a person. It can, but it can also touch the whole person. While many people use BDSM as a precursor to wild and exciting nookie, for many others BDSM is quite profound and reaches into areas of their lives beyond the sexual. It touches such things as their physiological, emotional, and even spiritual well-being.

It's worth then considering BDSM outside of mighty erections and tidal lubrication and looking at some of the many other areas of life which it can and does influence. Indeed, for this exercise we might want to actually consider BDSM as a tool which we can put to use to improve the general quality of life.

Some of the areas of life BDSM can effect include:

- Psychological

- Emotional

- Spiritual

- Physical

- Physiological

- Medical

- Relationships

Looking quickly at each of these...

Psychological condition and well-being

BDSM can create both opportunities for self-expression and opportunities to release pent-up energies and feelings which aren't easily available in a non-BDSM context. A slave may bare her back so her master can take out his frustrations on her and, at the same time, give her a solid and rewarding flogging. Someone who must stay in charge the whole day at work may find release with a dominant partner who deliberately takes charge and directs their life away from work. These sorts of behaviours can help provide useful outlets and psychological stability.

Emotional state and well-being

BDSM is often about lowering defences and being touched and affected by our partners. This can easily create emotional bonds between us. Also, the openness which BDSM requires for the most profound and satisfying experiences lends itself to providing intense emotional outlets for feelings of passion, sadness, and joy.

Spirituality

Spirituality is about being in touch with our inner selves. Because BDSM is frequently about honest self-expression, and because the intensity of some types of BDSM drives away pretence and leaves only raw feelings behind, our inner selves are often completely exposed and available to us, even if only for the duration of a scene. For some people, exposing their inner self to their partner can be the whole point of BDSM.

BDSM is also sometimes about peacefulness and this meditative aspect can appear in bondage scenes and in the quiet times after intense engagement with a partner.

Physical health and fitness

If nothing else in the health department, vigorous BDSM—such as heavy impact play or hoisting a bound submissive into the air as part of suspension bondage—is good for the cardiovascular system and helps build muscle. This applies both to tops and to bottoms.

There's more to fitness, of course, but the physical side of some forms of BDSM contributes to overall health. Additionally, because some BDSM activities involve risk of physical harm or infection—such as cutting, piercing, or heavy impact play which may break the skin (e.g., caning)—BDSM folk tend to be much more aware of such risks and know how to take steps to mitigate them. The benefits of this knowledge and of the safety-related habits we learn extend outside the dungeon.

Physiological well-being

To engage in many BDSM activities—even relatively benign ones such as a slave kneeling in front of her master—involves a certain level of flexibility, physical fitness, and an awareness of what things may impede one's ability to engage in BDSM. This means that many dedicated BDSM folk are very aware of their overall health, of the role of different types of food in their ability to perform, of the need to be well-rested, that drugs and alcohol negatively impact their BDSM, and so on.

Thus, BDSM folk can easily be more aware of and actively in control of their physiological condition than less active non-BDSM folk.

Medical condition

Following on from the above, to safely engage in BDSM means knowing and being respectful of any medical conditions which you or your partner might have. These can include:

- Susceptibility to asthma,

- Heart problems,

- Allergies,

- Epilepsy,

- High blood pressure,

- Low blood pressure,

- Diabetes,

- Haemophilia,

- Diarrhoea,

- Anosmia, or

- Cold, influenza or other infections which may influence breathing (e.g., a blocked nose).

Additionally, the effects of any medication being taken to treat a condition need to be known. For example, if someone is taking medication on whose bottle it says, "should not operate heavy machinery," they should not play.

Relationships

BDSM can provide opportunities for more closeness, more intimacy, and more honest and intense self-expression than is the norm outside of BDSM. This can be good for some relationships. Having in place strategies for dealing with BDSM-related problems which might crop up in a relationship often also means that these same strategies might help in the non-BDSM aspects of a relationship.

Read out to start the discussion

The great breadth and depth of BDSM means that there is the possibility that it can offer clues, guidance or influence in many, if not all, aspects of life. Not everyone wants this, of course. Some people look at BDSM as just a kinky detour on the road to sexual satisfaction, and some people look to it occupying just a small, isolated and safe part of their lives. It can however, be something which people embrace much more holistically. It can be the inspiration for growth, self development, well-being and happiness in many areas of their lives.

Some of these areas of life include:

- Psychological

- Emotional

- Spiritual

- Physical

- Physiological

- Medical

- Relationships

So. Is BDSM relevant to you in any or all of these areas? Are there any other areas in which your BDSM activities or relationships are involved?

Does your involvement in D&s or M/s help you be:

- A better member of society?

- A better boss?

- A better employee?

- A better parent?

Questions and remarks to nudge the discussion along

- What about work? Do any of the things you've learned or used from your BDSM experiences translate into the work environment?

- Are you more aware of what's going on around you in other relationships because of BDSM?

- How has BDSM improved you?

- The word "authenticity" is sometimes used in relation to BDSM. What does it mean and has BDSM helped you become more authentic?[1]

- Do you find BDSM challenging? Is this a good thing?

- Do you actually look for challenges in your life? Does BDSM provide you with the challenges you need?

- Are there any overall medical benefits to being into BDSM?

- Are there any overall psychological benefits to being into BDSM?

- How does BDSM impact your emotional life?

- How does BDSM effect self-awareness?

---

[1] See also topic 11 on page 57, *Authenticity*.

Topic 16

Spirituality

Presenter notes

In moments of ecstasy, it's not uncommon for people to talk to God as in, "Oh, god! Oh, God! OH, GOD!"

Behind the possible humour in this there can be a little grain of truth. In moments of excitement, intense emotions, or ecstasy, much of the surface of what we are is scratched away leaving our inner selves exposed. We might call this our soul, our spirit, or our inner being. Often the point of spirituality[1] is to bring someone into contact with this aspect of themselves and, here in BDSM, we have this happening just as a natural consequence of what we do.

Or perhaps it isn't just a consequence. Perhaps it is what we're trying to achieve anyway.

When we ask people what they're looking for from BDSM, the sorts of answers we get include:

- Hotter sex,

---

[1]Note that spirituality is also discussed in topic 15 on page 75, *Holistic BDSM*.

- Self actualisation,

- Uncovering their primal nature, or

- More profound experiences with their partner.

But aren't these all just different aspects of the same thing? Aren't we just talking about uncovering what's already inside the person?

While hotter sex is undoubtedly an admirable goal, perhaps a next step is to use BDSM, and the experiences it helps us create, to find our deeper selves.

BDSM experiences are often intense experiences, and it can be this intensity which pushes aside the habits, behaviours and ways of thinking which cover up our true selves thus helping us find these true selves. But a potential problem is that once the intensity is gone—such as after the end of a scene—the old habits, behaviours and ways of thinking will return.

Read out to start the discussion

Another place where you can find discussions about pain, suffering and deprivation are books about religion. They're usually focussed on the ideas of enlightenment, spirituality, self-discovery, and other high-minded concepts. This begs the question though: If enlightenment, spirituality and self-discovery are achievable through pain and suffering, why can't we get them through BDSM?

Or can we?

What is spirituality? Does it involve religion? Does it need to?

Are there different types of spirituality?

What can we achieve through BDSM?

Questions and remarks to nudge the discussion along

- Does spirituality need to involve an idea of a supreme being (such as a dominant[2])?

- Is pain a useful tool for achieving enlightenment? Does it need to be pain?

- How about submission? Is this a useful path to take to spirituality?

- Is spirituality just for submissives and slaves? What can a dominant or master get out of BDSM in the spirituality department?

- If we achieve some sort of enlightenment, awareness or understanding through BDSM, what can we do so that we don't lose it when we're not doing BDSM?

- Is surrender a part of this?

- So far, we've talked about using BDSM to achieve spirituality, but does it work the other way around: Does being spiritual help or enhance your BDSM activities or relationships? How so?

---

[2]This is attempted humour, though some BDSM folk involve worship as part of what they do so maybe this idea isn't so far off the track after all.

Topic 17

M/s, D&s, and our wider society

Presenter notes

One of the goals of talking about BDSM, both between ourselves and with others, is to demystify D&s and M/s relationships. Sometimes it isn't just people outside of BDSM who don't understand it, but also many of us on the inside don't always appreciate the scope and possibilities of BDSM.

Wider society, the folk who don't *do* BDSM and who know little about it, can find BDSM confusing and threatening. The idea of a man or a woman being subservient to another person on a voluntary basis[1] when it's not their occupation or employment is difficult to comprehend. Using pain or being locked in a cage to find ecstasy might be good theory in The Bible, but confronting it in real life or, worse, being confronted by someone who likes doing these things to others, can be downright scary and can be perceived as a threat by non-BDSMers to "normal" life.

Is this OK? I mean, is it OK for wider society to see BDSM like this?

---

[1]Or, at least, it looks voluntary, but that's another topic entirely.

Or should BDSM have a less hidden and better understood place in society?

In terms of wider society and acceptance, it's worth asking the question: Are there parallels between how BDSM is viewed by the wider community now and how the LGBT[2] community was viewed many years ago?

Is BDSM following along on the coat-tails of the LGBT community?

Read out to start the discussion

What is the place of BDSM in our wider society?

Parts of the LGBT community have long struggled to promote their acceptance by the wider community. We can see from events like the annual Folsom Street Fair in San Francisco and the Sydney Mardi Gras that this struggle has been somewhat successful. Even more, we've seen with the demise of the U.S. military's "Don't ask, don't tell" policy in 2011, with the legalisation of gay and lesbian marriage in many states and countries, and with smaller groups, associations and even schools coming out as "gay-friendly", that people are openly talking about it.

What about BDSM though?

To some extent, BDSM is getting a bit of a leg-up in terms of acceptance because it's commonly seen as a sexual proclivity and LGBT is precisely about sex... or, should I say, gender?

Is this where BDSM belongs, being seen as a not-too-distance cousin of LGBT?

Where should BDSM go?

---

[2]Lesbian, gay, bisexual and transgender

Questions and remarks to nudge the discussion along

- Community acceptance is one thing, but we can contrast this idea with the fact that it's common during many BDSM meetings and workshops to be encouraged not to even acknowledge our acquaintance of, or our friendships with other BDSM folk who we meet at these same workshops or meetings once we're back on the street in case someone sees.

Is public acceptance a direction that the BDSM community should go? Do we want acceptance so that we can be master and slave or dominant and submissive in public? Is there a plus side to this?

Is there a negative side to this?

- What is getting in the way of BDSM's acceptance by the wider community?

- Is there anything we, as BDSMers, can do or should be doing?

- Do members of the wider public view BDSM or BDSM folk as a personal threat? Do they feel they might get involved in something without wanting to? Is it uncertainty?

- Is there any similarity between how BDSM is perceived now and how LGBT was viewed in the past? What changed?

- What is abuse and how does it relate to all this?

In some legal jurisdictions, abuse is defined in terms of physical consequences (e.g., cuts or bruises) or physical actions (e.g., tying some up). This can be a judicial convenience along the lines of needing to have a certain amount of cash on you or else you can be declared by police to be a vagrant. It means that the police and courts, who represent precisely the wider community we're talking about, can easily deal with abusers, but how does this relate to BDSM where bruising and physical punishment can be a necessary component of a healthy relationship?

87

- Can or should wider society accept what we BDSM folk do to each other at times?

- Is just a subset of BDSM OK for wider society? Should parts of BDSM always remain in the shadows?

Topic 18

Foundations of BDSM as they apply to D&s and M/s

Presenter notes

According to yours truly (i.e., Peter Masters), there are three fundamental characteristics to all BDSM. They are:

1. Disparity or unequalness of power,

2. Penetration, and

3. Engagement.

Disparity of power—or unequalness of power—means that there is a deliberate effort by the people involved to recognise, impose and take advantage of a difference of power between themselves. This idea of it being deliberate is important because it's common for all sorts of people who interact with each other to be in positions of unequal power, skill or ability[1], but in BDSM it is

---

[1] Such as doctors and patients, lawyers and clients, police and criminals, and employers and workers.

the very deliberate exploiting of this difference productively for both people involved which makes it BDSM.

Having a difference in power is one thing, but in BDSM we use it to cause feelings and reactions in our partner. This applies equally to tops, masters and dominants just as much as it does to slaves, submissives and bottoms. The point is to *feel*, and the deeper the feelings and reactions, or the deeper the penetration, the more effective our BDSM is. If the feelings are completely superficial, then it's not really BDSM, it's probably just kinky.

Engagement is about our BDSM efforts being deliberately focused on the real person who is our partner. This has a lot to do with relationships. While wielding a mightly flogger a certain way might cause blubbery meltdowns in the average submissive, by learning the wants, needs and triggers of our particular partner we can direct our efforts at them personally and do things which we know will work for them personally. This is going to be far more profound.

Engagement is, in short, about being personal rather then being generic. Of course, the same applies in the other direction for submissives, slaves and bottoms who deliberately engage *their* masters, dominants and tops, rather than merely doing things which the average dominant will probably like.

If we agree that these three characteristics—disparity of power, penetration and engagement—are necessary foundations to all BDSM, how do they apply to D&s and M/s?

Where do we get or create an unequalness of power which we can exploit?

Power differences which can be useful in D&s or M/s come in different flavours. Here are a few:

- Drive or motivation to do or achieve something,
- A need to be in charge,
- A project—one of the dominant's or master's projects in which the slave or submissive can get involved,

- "Force of will" (whatever that is!),

- Physical strength—to physically dominate or overpower the slave or submissive,

- Intellect—to mentally or intellectually overpower or out-think the slave or submissive.

How do we get penetration?

For a start, penetration means deeply affecting. The word "deep" is a clue here because it means that the defences of the person being penetrated need to be lowered, and that means trust.

Continuing along the lines of a few of the suggestions above, the actual experience of physically dominating, or using main force to handle or manipulate a slave or submissive might be what penetrates a particular dominant. Or feeling that they are tools being used to achieve a useful and valuable goal may be what penetrates a particular slave or a submissive. Or merely being led or directed in everyday life may be comfortable and *right* for a submissive, and being the one taking the lead may be *right* for their dominant.

And how do D&s and M/s partners engage each other?

Engagement involves knowing your particular partner, so there's probably an element of time involved—time to learn what they like, what they need, what turns them on, and what turns them off.

Talking and asking questions is another important part of engagement. You shouldn't assume that you know what your partner likes or needs—this is the path to cookie-cutter BDSM. Instead, ask them; and if they don't ask you about your likes and needs, tell them.

Read out to start the discussion

There are common features to all of BDSM, to all activities, and to all BDSM relationships. When we recognise these we gain a way of understanding what it is that we need to put into our BDSM, and what we can get out of it.

In this workshop we look at these BDSM foundations and at how they apply to D&s and M/s relationships. Along the way we'll look at how to focus our efforts to get more bang for our BDSM buck, at what can go awry, and at what we can do to avoid the more common problems.

So. What do you consider to be the foundations of your own personal variety of BDSM, and do you think that any or all of them are foundations of BDSM in general?

Questions and remarks to nudge the discussion along

- What about power? What forms of power are in play in your relationship? What sorts of power work best for you?

- What about penetration? What is it that you do or say that has the deepest effect on your partner, and what is it that they do or say which has the deepest effect on you?

- What about engagement? Can we always do BDSM the same way with every partner we have? Why not? How do we learn what is the right or best way with a new partner?

- What effect do you have on your partner?

- What effect do they have on you?

- Here are some other things which are very common elements of BDSM. Are any of these fundamental for you?

    - Limits

    - Negotiation

- Safewords
- Sex
- Pain
- Bondage
- Teasing
- Service
- Training
- Authority
- Power
- Control
- TPE (Total Power Exchange)

- How does negotiation[2] enter into D&s or M/s? Does negotiation weaken a dominant's or master's position? Does it make it stronger?

- Safewords? Do they diminish D&s or M/s? Should they be *advisory words* instead? In other words, rather than saying "red" and meaning stop (which leaves control in the hands of the submissive), should it instead be that saying "red" means, "I'm having difficulty," so that the dominant can then choose what they do about it?

- What can diminish power? Or, what can diminish the effects of power or the power we actually feel? Decreased lust? What about when goals are reached or projects are completed? Do either of these signal a decrease in the feeling of involvement or penetration?

- What can diminish penetration? Trust issues? What sort of trust issues?

- What can diminish engagement? Distance? Assumptions (i.e., treating your partner as generic rather than as an individual)?

- How does a D&s or M/s relationship with a lot of engagement differ from one with little or no engagement?

---

[2]See also topic 10 on page 53, *Negotiation.*

- Is engagement necessary? Can D&s or M/s be satisfying without engagement?

- Does it need to be two-way?

Topic 19

Is saying "no" really control?

Presenter notes

Negotiation[1] is a frequent topic for newbies in BDSM. It's often about discussing with your partner the things to avoid such as agreeing that there'll be no intercourse, no leaving bruises, no scars, etc.

Another common BDSM topic is safewords. These are words or gestures used during a scene as signals. Common ones include "red" for stop and "yellow" for slow down. They're effective because instead of needing to get out of a hard-earned headspace to explain something to your partner, a simple word tells them when things are getting too much so that they can adjust their pace or stop what they're doing all together.

But in the way both of these topics are generally explored—negotiation and safewords, and particularly safewords—there's an implicit idea of "No!" Is this a good thing? I mean, is it right to be focusing on *not doing* rather on *doing*?

While saying "no" might be taking control, is it the right sort of control? Is it empowering to say "no"? Or is it really disempowering to say "no" because

---

[1] See also topic 10 on page 53, *Negotiation*.

you're actually chipping away at the things which you and your partner can do together? Note that I said "partner" here because it can equally be the top, dominant or master who says "no" to something just as much as it can be the bottom, submissive or slave. However, because the top, dominant or master is the one who is *doing*, instead of having to say "no" out loud they simply decide in themselves not to *do*.

Read out to start the discussion

Negotiation and safewords are important topics in BDSM. Negotiations are often about limits. Safewords are typically about ways to control or stop the action in a scene, with "red" being perhaps the most common safeword of all. "Red", of course, means stop immediately.

Both of these ideas—negotiation and safewords—are about saying "no". But because we're interested in D&s and M/s here, I'd like to ask the question: Is saying "no" really a way of acquiring control?

After all, a lot of what we talk about in M/s and D&s is control in one form or another. Isn't it the case though that by using "no" we are closing ourselves in or confining ourselves? That rather than creating possibilities, by saying "no" we are denying them?

Shouldn't we instead be looking at ways of saying "yes" to open ourselves up and move ourselves out of confinement?

Questions and remarks to nudge the discussion along

- Can a top, dominant or master say "no" or have a safeword? If so, how do they do it? How do they use their safeword?

- Is it the case that when you say "no" to anything that your partner will become cautious in future about doing anything at all?

- It's necessary to sometimes say "no", but how do you make sure that the way you say "no" to something actually opens doors rather than closes them?

- Should we be focusing more on finding ways to say "yes" during negotiations?

- Should we also be focusing more on making sure that we don't just have a "red" safeword but also have a just-as-important "green" one?

- Is there an ideal balance between "yes" and "no"?

Topic 20

Understanding roles

Presenter notes

We can define a role as a set of attitudes and behaviours which we adopt in a particular situation. In BDSM, our role—the attitudes and behaviours we adopt—determines how we interact with our partner. It is also a reflection of any wants or needs we might have and which we satisfy through our BDSM activities and relationships.

For example, being in a submissive role might mean that we can express and satisfy a need to serve or to be useful. Being in a slave role might mean we can surrender completely to our partner's authority and control. Being in a dominant role might mean we can satisfy a need to express primal aggression. And being in the role of a master might mean we can satisfy an urge to claim and exercise control over our partner.

We can also talk about a *primary* BDSM role. This would be the role which we adopt most of the time or which helps us satisfy our most important or driving wants and needs.

Some people only have a primary BDSM role and this never changes. Other people might have wants or needs which sometimes surface and which aren't necessarily compatible with what they see as their primary role. This doesn't mean the primary role needs to be abandoned, but maybe it does need to be put aside briefly from time to time. For example, if a dominant finds that occasionally being tightly bound by rope is important for his sanity or well-being, then he can briefly adopt the role of a bottom and be topped so that this need can be met while still being a dominant the rest of the time.

If it's a transient need, such as the abovementioned occasional need to be tied up, then it can be met with the person briefly adopting a different role for an occasional scene. If the want or need is more ongoing then it might be the case that the person has to have relationships with more than one person. For example, a slave to one person might also be in a satisfying relationship as someone else's dominant or top (as long as their master permitted it, of course).

As we see here, a role is not the person. The person can be the same, but the role they take on varies according to their needs and to their relationships with their partners.

We can also talk about *switches*. These are people who do change roles, possibly regularly, and who might not see themselves as having a fixed, primary role.

Importantly, the idea of wants or needs is closely tied to the idea of roles.

The role we adopt at any particular time needs to be understood in terms of:

- The wants and needs we hope to meet,
- How we meet them through that role's attitudes and behaviours,
- How our partner's wants and needs are met, and
- How one partner who normally sees us in one role is affected by seeing us in a different role.

There's an important point implicit in the above list, and that is that the role we adopt is going to directly affect which of our partner's wants and needs can be satisfied through us.

Read out to start the discussion

A role describes how we think and behave in a particular situation or with a particular person. If, for example, someone is keen to please their partner, we might say that they are a submissive. Someone else, who likes to see their partner writhing in orgasmic ecstasy, we might call a top.

Some common roles in BDSM are: top, bottom, dominant, submissive, master and slave.

How does a submissive differ from a slave?

How does a master differ from a top?

What other roles are there?

Questions and remarks to nudge the discussion along

- Roles to discuss. What attitudes and behaviours do each of the these roles have?

Top	Dominant	Owner
Bottom	Submissive	Property
Master	Trainer	*Mistress*
Slave	Trainee	*Switch*

- Many of the roles in BDSM complement other roles. For example, a top complements a bottom.

  How does a dominant complement a submissive? What does one do that the other needs, and vice versa?

- How does a master complement a slave?

- How does a top complement a bottom?

- Does our partner's role effect which of our wants or needs we can meet for ourselves?

- It's often the case that BDSM roles differ in term of authority. For example, a top generally needs to get the consent of their bottom each and every time they do something. A dominant instead might be able to do some things whenever they want without needing to ask their partner—they simply order their partner to comply at any time.

  Is this difference in authority true in all cases?

  - How is authority exercised with an owner and property compared to, say, a master and a slave?
  - Is authority relevant for a switch?
  - What authority does a top have in regard to their bottom?
  - What are the limits of authority for a dominant in regard to their submissive? How different is this compared to a master and their slave?

- Apart from gender, how does a mistress differ from a master?

Topic 21

The cost to a slave of disobeying

Presenter notes

A previous topic had to do with a story about a boat[1]. It was about a slave who built a boat with his friend. Then, sometime after completion of the boat, the slave's master ordered the slave to destroy this boat which he had co-built with his friend, and the slave did.

One of the things the boat story was intended to be about was respect[2].

Respect has to do with values, values other people have, rather than values we ourselves have.

In this light, this present topic looks at the cost to a slave of disobeying. That is, their values and what they suffer, rather than what other people might think about the ethics or morality of the situation the master might have put them in.

---

[1]Topic 14 on page 71, *The Boat.*
[2]See also topic 3 on page 19, *Respect.*

One cost to a slave is a fracturing or degrading of identity. For a slave, disobeying can be the first step on a path they don't want to be on—namely, second-guessing their master. We might say that for a slave surrendering to their condition is the goal they aim for. Note that I said *condition*, and not *master*. If they passionately and deeply need to be slave, then achieving that surrender establishes and provides a solid foundation for their identity. If they need to question that foundation, it destabilises it and necessarily devalues them in their own eyes as a slave.

Beyond this, we can say as a generalisation that no one becomes a slave just to do what they're told. They look for more than that out of it. It might provide mental or emotional contexts in which they can function best. It might be that a slave needs that constraint to help them focus on achieving goals. Losing their slave identity (or losing the master/mistress they trust and with whom they can be slave) can have a high price in terms of being able to function.

Third, when a slave is a member of a BDSM group or community then the cost of disobeying can be ejection from the group and the consequent loss of friends and other benefits which membership of the group affords. Being part of such a group provides a very big motivation to obey because the cost of not doing so can be loss of friends, loss of community, loss of associated benefits, and isolation.

All of these things weigh on a slave when they receive an order which is questionable and they will look for ways of justifying obedience such as psychological denial or projection: "master must know something I don't", "it's not really that bad", "it's not my responsibility", "he'll understand", etc. Such justifications are probably not good things anyway because they introduce mental gymnastics in the slave which take away from the M/s.

Read out to start the discussion

Is it OK for a slave to disobey their master?

Are there particular situations where they should disobey?

Does anything break when a slave disobeys their master?

Does trust in their master get damaged in such circumstances? Can this be repaired?

For some slaves, being slave is part of their self-identity. What happens to this identity if they feel forced to disobey?

Questions and remarks to nudge the discussion along

- What happens if an order is completely ethical for the master but unethical for the slave?

  Do a slave's own values and standards get subjugated to the master's?

- Should a slave second-guess their master?

- Should a master provide a way for a slave to question the ethics of an order, or should it be the job of the slave simply to obey and resolve any contradictions themselves?

- Should a slave obey an order they find questionable just to prevent their relationship with their master from breaking?

Topic 22

Relationships - making (good) and breaking (bad)

Presenter notes

BDSM is not always famous for long-term relationships. It is instead often seen as just consisting of occasional intense encounters between two people with long periods of no BDSM in between. But whether you're in, or interested in, a long-term relationship, or whether you're pursuing a quick scene with someone you've just met at a play party, we're still talking relationships.

Compatibility in terms of wants and needs is a big factor in relationships. For example, if a submissive is into heavy rough-handling (i.e., physical domination) and she meets a dominant who is into micromanagement, they may not have enough in common to be able to satisfy each other. On the other hand, when a dominant with a more hands-off approach meets up with a self-motivated, service-oriented submissive then they may be able to work together very well indeed.

Another factor is frequency and strength of needs. If a submissive only needs to feel the firm hand of a dominant every week or so and she tries to set up house with a dominant with daily needs, then someone is probably going to end up not completely happy.

So even with the best of intentions things may not work out between two committed D&s or M/s folk. It can get even more problematic when one or both are not being completely open and honest with their partner, when they have selfish or hidden motives, or when they simply don't understand themselves well enough to know what they need versus what they merely desire.

Indeed, for D&s and M/s to work well, it behoves[1] each person to be aware of the wants and needs of both themselves *and* their partner and to work towards ensuring that all of them are met.

Read out to start the discussion

It's common (and easy) for BDSM folk to focus on the mechanical side of BDSM—on scenes, implements, dungeons, and so on. But the relationship side of things is vital, and even if we're talking about short scenes at a play party, we still need to relate to the person we're with even if we may not be ever seeing them again.

Relating has to do with ensuring that we know which of our wants and needs we're hoping to meet through our partner, which of their wants and needs they hope to meet through us, and then working to make sure we both get what we need.

So, there are some questions we can ask:

Why have a relationship? Can't you just treat the person you're playing with like meat, or just treat them like a flogger which happens to have some man attached to the handle, especially if you just meet them at a play party?

What are the roles of personal responsibility, maturity, and self-awareness for a dominant or master? What about these roles for a submissive or slave?

How does a 24/7 D&s or M/s relationship work and keep on being satisfying?

---

[1] Such an under-appreciated word! It means having a duty or responsibility to do something.

Questions and remarks to nudge the discussion along

- What's the difference between a short-term D&s or M/s relationship, and a long-term one? Can you engage in D&s or M/s with someone you meet at a play party just during the party? What limitations are there on such a short-term D&s or M/s encounter?

- What can't you do in short-term D&s or M/s?

- What differences are there between a BDSM relationship and a non-BDSM relationship?

- Are there different sorts of D&s relationship? What sort do you need personally? What sort of D&s wouldn't work for you at all?

- How can you have a powerful scene at a party with someone you have just met? What's actually going on here? Can you really have a strong connection with someone you just met?

- What factors are important for you in determining whether someone would be a good D&s or M/s partner?

- What's the difference between a want and a need? How can you tell if something is really a need for you or your partner?

- What can go wrong in a relationship?

    - Unreasonable expectations?
    - Lack of knowledge about yourself (which you then can't communicate to your partner)?
    - Growing apart?
    - Losing interest?
    - Dominants pretending to be infallible?
    - Excessive self-sacrifice by a submissive?

- What poor reasons can someone have for getting involved in a BDSM relationship?

- Self-worth issues?
- Avoiding responsibility (for submissives)?
- Easy way to get sex (for horny young male "doms")?
- Selfishness?

- What can else can go wrong?

  - What can you do to fix it? (Clue: communication very often helps)

Topic 23

Control of your partner

Presenter notes

One of the fundamental ideas in much of BDSM is that of one person—a dominant or master—controlling their partner—a submissive or slave. Smoothly taking control of someone, using them, and then neatly handing control back when you're done (if appropriate) is not always easy and the processes involved in short-term and long-term control of another person are rarely discussed in BDSM manuals.

There are actually four steps involved in taking control of someone. In short:

1. The submissive (or slave) internally, and possibly unconsciously, makes control over some aspect of themselves available,

2. The dominant (or master) signals that they are taking up the offer,

3. The submissive relinquishes control to the dominant, and

4. The dominant accepts and starts using that control.

The control I'm talking about here can be anything about a submissive or slave. It can be what they wear or how they speak. It can be about the dominant grabbing them by the scruff of the neck and guiding/pushing them down into a kneeling position. It can be about sending them out on an errand. It can be about sex—how, when, and with whom they do it. In sum, it can be about anything imaginable that you can do to them or instruct them to do.

But before a dominant can take control over some aspect of them, the submissive has to be prepared to hand over that control (step 1). This doesn't mean that they actually do hand over control at this point, but they do prepare themselves to do so. While they're waiting for someone (e.g., a dominant) to take up the offer (step 2), they continue to exercise the control themselves such as deciding when and with whom to have sex, what errands to do, etc.

Once a dominant signals they are taking up control, the submissive surrenders it (step 3) *and stops asserting it themselves*. In other words, if a submissive surrenders control to a dominant over what errands they do, they stop doing errands until the dominant instructs them to do so.

Finally, the dominant starts using the control they have claimed (step 4).

There are a number of places where this process can go awry. For example, if a dominant thinks that a submissive is ready for him to control by the scruff of the neck (step 1) and the submissive actually isn't, then the dominant will grab her by the neck (attempting step 2) and will get a surprise when she doesn't yield.

The idea behind this workshop is exploring the steps listed above, and also looking at:

- Prerequisites of control,
- What control a dominant can have,
- Usefully and productively doing something with control,
- How a dominant can unintentionally lose control,
- Handing back control when the dominant is done with it, and
- What [else] can go wrong.

For more detail on the topic, read my book on the subject, *The Control Book*.

Read out to start the discussion

In the BDSM worlds of D&s and M/s, authority, power, and control are the coin of the realm, the currency which we trade and use to make good things happen. In this topic we're going to look at the final one of these: control.

Even if we have authority and power, taking control, using it effectively, and handing it back when we're done (an often neglected step!) are not always well understood.

The process of taking control, and later handing it back when we're done, involves four steps:

1. Offering control - the submissive or slave makes control over some aspect of themselves available,

2. Taking up the offer - the dominant or master signals they are taking up the offer,

3. Relinquishing control - the submissive or slave actually surrenders the control, and

4. Accepting and asserting the control - the dominant or master takes up and starts using the control.

Do these sound right to you?

What sorts of control do these apply to? Are these steps universally applicable?

Why take control? What's the point?

What happens when a dominant tries to take control that isn't offered? Do they get the equivalent of a slap in the face?

Questions and remarks to nudge the discussion along

- What prevents your master or dominant controlling you more than they do? Is it that they don't care to, or is it that you won't hand over more control? If the latter, why?

- What's involved in handing back control? When and why do you do this?

- What happens to a submissive or slave if their dominant or master doesn't hand back control when they're done with it?

  As a concrete example, suppose a master tells his slave not to go to the toilet without his permission, and then some time later he goes away somewhere without rescinding or changing the order. What happens? Does the slave or submissive explode?

- Can a master or dominant lose control after they've got it? Can a submissive or slave take it back? When can this happen?

- Can a master delegate control to someone else?

- Go through each of the four steps above and ask your group if they can list one or more problems which might occur at each step. For example, a situation where a submissive who has offered up control and thinks a dominant is taking it up, but the dominant has no such intention (i.e., there was a communication problem or misunderstanding).

Topic 24

Starting a D&s or M/s relationship

Presenter notes

Starting a D&s or M/s relationship has some things in common with starting a non-BDSM relationship. There are also some things which are unique to BDSM. In this topic, we're interested in the things which are unique to BDSM relationships.

For a start, most people have some general idea about how a non-BDSM relationships is going to start and evolve because these get portrayed a lot in movies, on TV, in books, and in magazines. We also get to talk about them with other people, such as at work with colleagues.

BDSM relationships, on the other hand, are not so well-known and for someone looking to have a D&s or M/s relationship for the first time, there will be many things that they won't know and which will possibly surprise them.

For example, common interests—such as shared political or religious views, same attitudes towards having children, or same interests in food or entertainment—are usually very important in non-BDSM relationships, but in

D&s and M/s this may not be the case. Instead there often needs to be a focus on exercising authority and control. How do you develop and maintain this focus long-term? Who is going to teach you?

Boundaries can also be a new problem. If you're a slave, how much influence should your master have over your financial affairs such as your job, your retirement planning or your insurance? What about your health care choices? Should your master have any influence on your other relationships, such as with friends or family? These are questions which won't arise in the non-BDSM world.

Communication, openness and honesty (both with your partner and with yourself) are often the biggest keys here. Many problems can develop because of wrong expectations, and talking can help keep these to a minimum. A dominant or master doesn't lose authority by saying they don't know. They instead often lose it by trying to fumble their way forward in ignorance. A slave or submissive often looks to their partner to be in charge, not necessarily to be all-knowing.

Read out to start the discussion

How do you go from the first stirring that you'd either like to be kneeling at another's feet, or that you'd like to have someone kneeling at yours, to actually being in this situation with another person?

How do you chart a course from being two separate people who think they might be able to do something together, to being a fully-functional, committed D&s or M/s couple, regularly and consistently engaging each other, communicating smoothly and often without words, and confidently knowing how each other ticks?

If you're looking for a D&s or M/s relationship now, what is it that you want exactly? What are you wanting from your future partner? What are you prepared to give?

If you're already in a D&s or M/s relationship, what is it that you get out of the relationship beyond what a non-BDSM relationship might give you?

How do you meet a D&s or M/s partner, i.e., your future master, slave, submissive or dominant?

116

How do you know that they're *the one*?

Is there anything you need to do before you try and set yourself up with a D&s or M/s partner, especially the first time?

Questions and remarks to nudge the discussion along

- What boundaries are important? If you're a dominant or master, what areas of your submissive's or slave's life would you not try to influence?

    - Their relationships with other friends or family?
    - Their future financial security?
    - Their job?
    - Any medical treatment they may need? Health care planning?

- Is your BDSM going to take place just in either planned or impromptu scenes? Scenes can be times of great focus, but they aren't necessarily all there is. What about the rest of the time?

- What expectations are reasonable?

- What expectations are unreasonable?

- If you don't work at maintaining the D&s or M/s "edge" in a relationship, it risks slowly drifting into just kinky sex. How do you recognise that this is happening? How do you stop it? What can you do?

- What are good goals for a D&s or M/s relationship? Should you actually have goals? What happens to the relationship if and when you achieve all the goals?

- Is there a potential problem of passion fading? How do you keep the interest up?

- What other problems might occur?

- What's actually required in a D&s or M/s relationship for it to succeed (emphasis on *D&s* and *M/s*), and what's irrelevant window dressing?

- What's the role of authority in your relationships?

  - What about power?
  - And what about control?

- What does your D&s or M/s partner need from you?

- What do you need from them?

- How do you say "I don't know" while still staying in charge?

- What's the role of discipline and/or correction for you?

- Trust can be vital. It has a very big role in bringing down barriers and defences, and in allowing engagement. Specifically, it's important to allowing the engaging of sensitive parts of ourselves which we often try to protect.

  Trust means that if you get the most out of your D&s activities while dressed as a chicken with Rick Dee's Disco Duck playing loudly on the stereo, then you can say so without fearing being diminished or devalued because of it.

  What do you need to develop trust?

- How do you ensure good communication? In D&s and M/s, the slave or the submissive can feel it's inappropriate to express their thoughts or feelings, or that it's inappropriate to be critical. They may feel that it's not their place to do so to such an extent that they end up suffering unreasonably because they won't speak up. How do you ensure they do? Should they keep a diary which you read? Should there be set times (e.g., weekly) when they can freely speak their mind?

Topic 25

Ritual and structure in D&s and M/s relationships

Presenter notes

Of course, no dominant actually dominates 24 hours a day, 7 days a week. Sometimes they're asleep. Sometimes they're watching TV. Sometimes they might even be at work. The point is that while the two of you might be in what you could call a 24/7 relationship, the actual D&s or M/s really occurs only at intervals. The rest of the time, D&s or M/s aren't happening.

It's not just the dominants who aren't dominating 24/7. Sometimes a submissive is concerned with other things, such as their work or an exciting visit to their proctologist. Or they may have non-BDSM friends who they meet, or they might be visiting with their parents, brothers or sisters. Or they might be doing something else completely mundane which doesn't have anything to do with D&s. And even if their dominant happens to be physically present with them, they might be watching TV, or doing their tax return or something else which distracts them from being dominant.

So in a D&s or M/s relationship what you get are periods of actual mastery, slavery, domination or submission occurring between the two people involved, followed by often long intervals without.

When we're talking about D&s and M/s, what we're usually referring to is the exercise and experience of authority, power and control. What do we do to keep these magical D&s and M/s juices running when we're not actually interacting D&s-wise or M/s-wise with our partner?

This is where ritual and structure come in.

Ritual involves doing things in a certain way. For example, a slave might bow down in front of her master each time she enters a room he's in. We might cynically say that ritual complicates things without making them more efficient or effective. In the case of kissing feet, the ritual simply makes it more time consuming for the slave to go into a room and maybe life'd be simpler if she simply waited for her master to go somewhere else so that she could go into the room without mucking about with his shoes.

But ritual isn't about efficiency and effectiveness. It's about reinforcing the dynamic that exists between two BDSM folk. If a submissive is tasked with making the communal bed each morning, she might kneel to tuck the sheets in, and this act of kneeling can pleasantly remind her of her station in the relationship.

Structure, on the other hand, is less about doing things in certain ways, and more about doing things as directed by the master or dominant. For example, a master might order his slave to rise in the morning 30 minutes before he does, to tidy herself and make herself pleasing to look at, and to prepare the breakfast table. In this it isn't so much about the way she does what she's been told, but the outcomes. The point is that she has orders to follow which give her the awareness of control, even when her master is still asleep.

Read out to start the discussion

When you are in a D&s or M/s relationship, a certain amount of pleasure and satisfaction comes from interacting directly with your partner. For example, this can be when a dominant takes charge of and directs his submissive in some activity, or when a slave is performing some act of personal service for his or her mistress.

The point about these things is that they directly involve each partner in the relationship. They directly interact with each other. Indeed, this sort of one-on-one interaction can be most powerful.

120

But what happens when these two partners aren't physically in the same place, such as when one or both are at work. If they can't interact one-on-one any more does the D&s or M/s stop?

What about when they are, say, living together but happen to be in different rooms of the house? Can and does the D&s and M/s continue when they're out of each other's sight?

And if they happen to be sitting in front of the TV, both engrossed in some movie, is the D&s or M/s still there? If it is, is it dormant waiting for one or the other to do something that involves their partner, such as for the master to instruct his slave to get him a drink?

In sum, is there something which keeps D&s or M/s happening when both people involved aren't actually and intentionally interacting with each other?

Is ritual part of the answer?

What about structure or standing orders imposed by the dominant or master, such as how to do certain things?

Questions and remarks to nudge the discussion along

- This topic is about rituals and structure in BDSM. We can maybe say that ritual is about doing things in certain ways, and that structure is about things to do and standing orders to follow. Is this a good way of differentiating between the two?

- Structure can be about a slave or submissive learning their master's preferences—such as in food, drink, or clothing—or learning their master's ethical and moral values and then using these to determine how they, the submissive or slave, should act when their master is not around.

  Beyond what's listed below, what else could be considered structure?

  – How the slave or submissive should dress,
  – How the slave or submissive should behave towards others, and
  – What food or drink to prepare or order for their master.

- What standing orders do you (or your submissive) have?

- Should you, or do you, as a master or dominant, have your own rituals or structure which support your relationship with your partner?

- What rituals do you have which support your D&s or M/s? Are there any you do just in the bedroom? When you're out in public? When you're somewhere private but with your clothes on?

- Are there any rituals you follow which "put you in the mood"? For example, in the world of topping and bottoming, when a top is unpacking their toybag prior to a scene, or when they put on their leathers, this often starts to put them in the mood for play. Is there anything similar in your D&s or M/s?

- What do you do when your partner isn't around which helps you *feel* the D&s or M/s which exists between you?

- When you perform your rituals, do you have an image of your partner in your mind as you do them?

- When we're looking for definitions, is it fair to say that ritual comes from the submissive or slave, and that structure comes from their master or dominant?

Appendices

Definitions

BDSM   A compound acronym representing the terms Bondage and Discipline, Dominance and Submission, and Sadism and Masochism

BDSMer   Someone who practices BDSM

BDSM-land A place, state of mind, or relationship in which BDSM is practiced

D&s   Dominance and submission

LGB   Lesbian, gay and bisexual

LGBT   Lesbian, gay, bisexual and transgender

M/s   Mastery and slavery

Mind-fuck Deliberately being obscure, opaque, confusing or contradictory to create uncertainty, insecurity or doubt

Nookie   Sexual intercourse

Old Guard Usually refers to the gay, biker subculture which began to appear in the USA in the 1940's. This lead to, or influenced, leather, S&M, and eventually BDSM.

Safeword   An agreed word or phrase which, when used during a scene, immediately brings activity to a halt. For example, a submissive reaching their pain limit may say the word "red" to let their top know they need to stop. A safeword like "red" is used instead of a word like "stop" because in the throes of passion a submissive might keep saying "stop" when they are really having a fantastic time.

Scene   1.   One or more connected activities in which two partners engage, these activities having a clear start and end. For example, a bondage scene where the dominant ties up his submissive and then flogs her, or a punishment scene where a submissive undresses, leans over a low table, and is then caned on the buttocks.

2.   A particular community of BDSM folk.   For example, the local bondage scene, or the local under-30s scene, etc.

S&M   Sadism and masochism

Sub-space A feeling of floating or detachment which can occur during some BDSM experiences. It's often considered a desirable goal of some activities. It can be a *high* for some people, and it is sometimes accompanied by the release of neurochemicals in the brain, particularly when pain is involved such as through caning, flogging, etc.

About the author

Peter Masters was born in Sydney in 1958 and is not dead yet. He first discovered an interest in controlling fine females in his early teens. For reasons probably related to ads on the back pages of comic books of the time his first interest in this area took the form of hypnosis. This was for the totally venal reason of getting laid. It was, however, a surprise that so many women would allow themselves to be hypnotised when the consequences to their nether regions seemed quite obvious.

This interest in hypnosis and sex led eventually, some 30 or so years later, to the book *Look Into My Eyes*, a handbook for using hypnosis to make sex very interesting based on his experience with many partners and trances too numerous to even guess at.

Subsequently he learned that many women—even some casual acquaintances and professional colleagues—seem to respond quite well to an authoritative stance and many were attracted to this. Thus his entry into the world of BDSM was through dominance and submission and this remains his main passion. Knots and floggers were never a great interest, but if getting close to a naked woman required either then he was always ~~desperate enough~~ prepared to make the effort.

The exploration of authority, power and control aspects of dominance and submission with partners, friends and others led to a second book, *The Control Book*, which is about taking, giving, building, reinforcing, relinquishing and losing control of someone. Peter has run discussion groups on dominance and submission, given workshops and presentations on BDSM and BDSM-related topics over the years and, of course, writes the occasional book on BDSM.